# FAST WITH PAIGE

*Health & Healing Practices for Forever Freedom*

WRITTEN BY PAIGE DAVIDSON

WITH KIM SMITH

An Unbelievable Freedom Book

Credits:

Clagett Photography
Elizabethtown, KY

"Hair by Shannon"
Hair and make-up, Shannon Newton
Frankfort, KY

Polish'd Nail Spa
Nails, Chasity Hawkins
Lexington, KY

---


Designed and formatted by Eled Cernik.
ISBN-13: 978-1-954248-00-7

# DEDICATION

*To my faithful and loving Mother, Vivian Jackson, who knew my calling was to be a health coach years before I did. You have always known my heart!*

*And to the compassionate Linda Fentress, Compass Christian Counseling, who gently and lovingly guided me in understanding that what I thought was a weight loss journey was actually a spiritual journey with physical healing. You helped me to allow God to change the trajectory of my life, and I am ever grateful.*

*I keep fighting voices in my mind that say I'm not enough*
*Every single lie that tells me I will never measure up*
*Am I more than just the sum of every high and every low?*
*Remind me once again just who I am, because I need to know,*

*You say I am loved when I can't feel a thing*
*You say I am strong when I think I am weak*
*And You say I am held when I am falling short*
*And when I don't belong, oh You say I am Yours*
*And I believe, oh I believe,*
*What you say of me.*
*I believe*

YOU SAY
LAUREN DAIGLE

# Table of Contents

# Welcome from Kim

Greetings, Freedom Seekers!

New adventures are on the horizon for Unbelievable Freedom Books, but in the meantime, I'm honored to present our newest author, Paige Davidson. She's here to teach what she learned on her spiritual journey with physical healing, all of which resulted in a total transformation.

Paige's story is my story, in many ways. There is shame and discouragement, seeking and struggling, overcoming and triumphing. Like me and many others, Paige recognizes that the "inner work" needed to occur in order for any health plan or practice to be successful. Like me and many others, Paige sees fasting as both a spiritual and a physical practice.

While the full story is vast, we've set things up to give you enough inspiration and information to move into ACTION.

This book is organized as follows:

- Part 1: Fast with Paige PLATFORM - Fasting as the Transformation Foundation
- Part 2: Fast with Paige PRACTICES - Healing Habits that Build Up
- Part 3: Fast with Paige "PLUS" - Additional Resources and Extra Inspiration

Step forward in faith. Believe and take action. That's where the real magic happens.

Enjoy Your Life,
Kim

Paige Davidson encourages you to consult your healthcare provider before making any health-related change. This guide cannot be used as a replacement for consultation with your healthcare provider and does not constitute medical advice.

# Welcome from Paige

As I anxiously awaited my first visit with a Christian therapist, I felt like I was going to hyperventilate. My palms were sweaty, and my mind was racing. Which humiliating part of my story would we discuss first? Which painful things was I going to have to reveal? How was this going to help me with what I had battled for years: I could not control food; it controlled me. It drove my mood, my beliefs about myself, and especially my actions.

When would I feel comfortable enough to express how my battle with food had been amplified by years' worth of humiliations, sleights, and either being ignored completely or overtly ridiculed because I was morbidly obese?

What words could express my nausea and deepening sense of dread before every job interview, knowing I'd likely be forced - once again - to endure the devastation of being passed over for jobs for which I was highly qualified. The interviewer's eyes continually betrayed their thoughts, "You don't have enough self-control not to be fat. How can I trust you to be able to do this job?"....or worse?

I still flinch at the memory of ordering lunch at a fast food drive-thru, my order interrupted by a car full of teenage boys driving by, hurling trash at my car, cruelly laughing and screaming "Way to go, fatso! Pig out and get even fatter!!" Not only did the restaurant employee hear it, but customers heard it as well. The poor drive-thru girl stammered and said how sorry she was that had happened. I just could not face her; my face was flushed with embarrassment and hot tears as I fled in humiliation. That same feeling of humiliation haunts me to this day whenever I recall this event. How can I possibly make this therapist understand how degraded I felt that day?

The looming fear of having to discuss these painful situations suddenly felt crushing, and I desperately wanted to get out of there.

Just in the nick of time, Linda, the therapist, came out and greeted me with a warmth and kindness that was palpable. I intuitively trusted her, and knew that I was going to be safe in her hands.

She asked, "So, Paige, why have you come to see me today?" My nervousness evaporated and I opened up. "Linda, there is something really wrong with me. I don't know if I have an eating disorder, a food addiction, or maybe OCD related to food. Whatever it is, I've just got to get it figured out, and solve the problem once and for all, because I can't continue on this way any longer."

As we talked, the first shameful memory that I disclosed was that as a child, I snuck food into my room, hiding and eating it when I wanted, because I didn't like being told what I could and couldn't eat. As a young teenager, I attended a commercial weight-loss center (this was the first of the many, many times I joined, then soon quit, this program over the next 40+ years, my self-esteem falling each time I quit). As time went on, I attended every commercial weight-loss center there was. I lost weight each time, but I lost a little bit of myself, too. I would hang on until I could no longer tolerate the restrictions, limitations, rules around food, counting, logging, and even taking shots with needles and prescription medicines. The inevitable was always a sense of failure and regaining of the weight I had worked so hard to lose. I never once loved myself through the process. Just the opposite, I berated myself for being so weak.

After years of yo-yo dieting and finding myself at 315 pounds, I was desperate and defeated enough to undergo Roux-N-Y gastric bypass surgery in 2000. I lost 150 pounds over the next year and a half. However, my "success" was brief. I only maintained that loss for four years, and then, as I slowly returned to my old eating habits, the inevitable weight gain resumed, along with the shame, guilt, and crushing sense of failure.

The cycle of dieting resumed, and the extremes I went through to lose weight, each time hoping against hope that this one would finally change things, led me in a spiral of shame and failure. When I finally accepted the only thing diets ever did for me was cause me to gain weight, I officially declared "No more diets, ever!" However, I was back up to 249 pounds and in an absolute panic about that. I knew I needed to do something, but I knew it was not found in another diet. I decided to try the only thing there was left to try, counseling.

The journey with Linda began the course that changed my life. Through exploration, we unpacked the baggage I was carrying, and with her professional expertise, she confirmed I did not have an eating disorder. We did heavy work together to allow me to lighten this load I carried around regarding my weight and self-control around food.

Alongside the work I was investing into my spiritual and mental wellness, I was introduced to the practice of intermittent fasting (IF). I was resistant at first, because I was "never dieting again"; however, upon further and deeper understanding of the practice, I realized it was not a diet but a health tool that promotes healing and wellness, along with a sense of management around food and a side benefit of weight loss. My physical state was suffering; plantar fasciitis and Achilles tendonitis left me limping and barely able to walk. Despite myself, IF piqued my curiosity.

My journey was forever changed by the book *Delay, Don't Deny* by Gin Stephens. With Linda's awareness and approval, I began to explore the practice of IF, with the primary desire to heal my painful conditions. Within two weeks, I was no longer limping. Although still in pain, I could walk normally! Within six months, I was completely pain-free. And, to my shock, I had lost over 50 pounds while eating without rules or regulations around food. Further proof of the benefits I experienced are:

- I completely healed the inflammation in my feet.
- I no longer suffered from obstructive sleep apnea.
- My chronic depression lifted, and I was able to discontinue one medication and greatly reduce another.
- I have lost 110 pounds.
- All my health markers - blood pressure, blood glucose, cholesterol, BMI and weight - are all in the healthy, normal range after practicing IF for over a year and a half.
- I have become a fitness walker, walking 4-6 miles a day.
- My success story was featured in Woman's World magazine, and I was pictured on the cover (see resources section).
- I began a program to earn an Integrative Health Coach certification.
- I started a virtual business as an IF Consultant and Mentor.

Since you are reading this book, you might relate to some of my experiences as an obese, or morbidly obese, person. My story is filled with broken pieces, humiliation, repeated failures and terrible habits and choices. Does this resonate with you? If so, please know there is hope for your future!

Because my story also includes a major comeback, peace and joy in my food choices and my life, and a lifestyle shift that finally allowed me to reach long-term health and weight-loss goals. And, this absolutely can be part of your story, as well.

I want to welcome you! I'm so glad you are here and ready to regain control of your eating habits, your health and wellness, and your future. Are you ready to experience true contentment, peace, and joy in your life?

Repeat after me: I CAN do this!!!

PART ONE

# Fast with Paige PLATFORM - Fasting as the Transformation Foundation

# Introduction-Diet Freedom

My unsuccessful dieting history is a painful one. Can you relate? However, there is one experience I always dread sharing, and that's a sense of having failed at the 'ultimate' weight loss solution, gastric bypass surgery. How does one expose such searing shame, disillusionment, and humiliation? I will never forget my surgeon saying, "We can operate on your stomach, but we can't operate on your brain." And yet there was no assistance with changing my thoughts along with my stomach.

Gastric bypass surgery was the most extreme measure I took, but it was one of a litany. Ultimately, I spent over 40 years trying every type of intervention you can imagine, all in a quest to lose weight and keep it off. I was even called a "professional dieter" by the owner of one weight loss establishment, when he heard all the different diets and weight loss businesses I had tried, always unsuccessfully. During one of my frequent internet searches for "the answer", I stumbled upon the following:

*It is not just about losing the weight. It is about losing the mindset and lifestyle that got you there in the first place.*

This really got my attention. What did mindset and lifestyle have to do with being able to lose weight and keep it off? Wasn't losing weight about what you eat and doing rigorous exercise to go along with it? This was a question I brought to my therapist early on in our work together.

Over the last year and a half of my life as I lost 110 pounds, I learned that shifts in mindset and lifestyle have EVERYTHING to do with losing weight and keeping it off. I learned that we have power over our mindset, and there are two kinds of lifestyles: the kind you choose, and the kind that chooses you. I became empowered to change my mindset and choose what kind of lifestyle I was going to live, and this workbook will guide you to do the same.

Since this is a workbook about how to lose a significant amount of weight and keep it off permanently, the first question you have is undoubtedly, "What kind of diet do I have to do?"

Here is the surprising answer – none. You are not going to diet. In fact, you are never going to do another diet, ever! The reason is simple; diets DO NOT work!

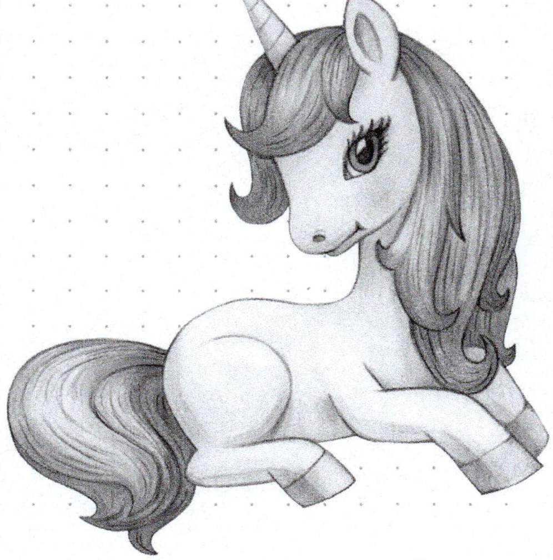

- Dieting takes away your ability to be an intuitive eater and make the best decisions for yourself; it puts the expertise and responsibility outside of you, forcing you to place all of your focus on external rules or a specific regimen.
- Bio-individuality, a scientifically proven concept, proves there is no one right way for every person to eat. We are all unique, and one person's food is another person's poison. Many factors influence which food choices are right for us as individuals: our general health, age, values, background, preferences, potential food sensitivities, schedule, activity levels and even who we spend time with.
- Dieting leaves you feeling frustrated and guilty when you can't follow the stringent rules of the diet perfectly, leaving you vulnerable to unhealthy eating patterns.

What if you set aside all your complicated diets with their rules, food lists, counting points, calories, macros, and micros, and just tried the simplest and most effective path toward health?

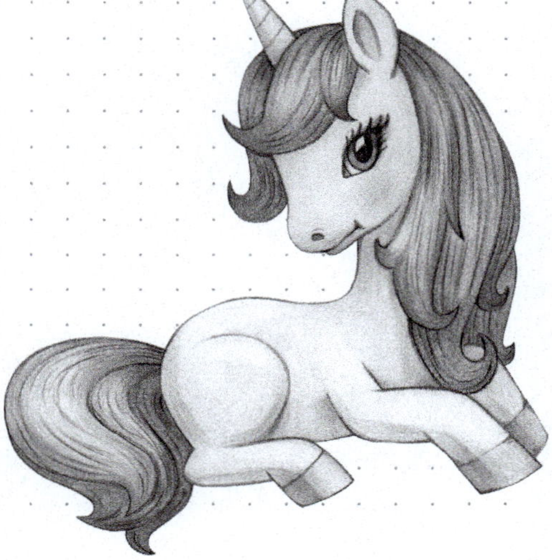

# *The WHAT of Intermittent Fasting

Intermittent fasting is an eating pattern where you cycle between periods of eating and periods of clean fasting.

Intermittent fasting tells you WHEN to eat, not WHAT to eat. Enjoy the foods that you choose to eat within your eating window.

Intermittent fasting is not a diet, but a pattern of eating. For example, you may choose to follow the 16/8 protocol. This means you clean fast for 16 hours and eat during an 8-hour period.

Intermittent fasting (IF) is a specific way of managing your food each day. I was fortunate to discover IF early in my work with my therapist, and I practiced IF as I lost 110 pounds and reached maintenance. I'll always live an IF lifestyle. While this book isn't just about IF, it's the foundation that will ENABLE you to become the person who will reach your health and weight loss goals.

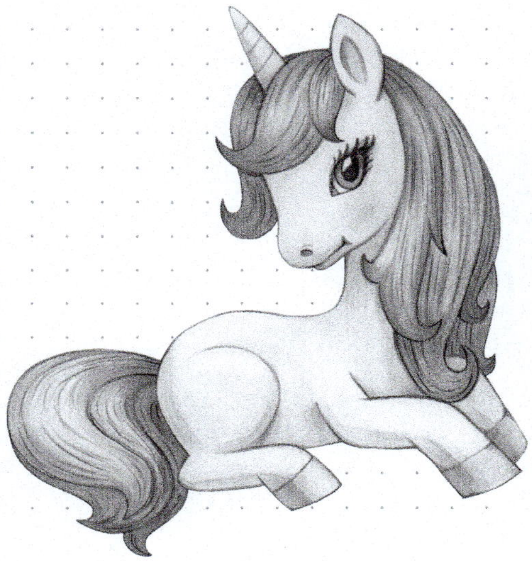

# *The WHY of Intermittent Fasting?

IF is an incredibly healthy lifestyle, with the wonderful side effect of weight loss. It has myriad health benefits, including*:

- combats hyperinsulinemia
- preventing prevents and reversing reverses metabolic syndrome
- can prevent and even reverse Type 2 Diabetes
- anti-inflammatory, a dangerous condition for the body
- shows promise for those with autoimmune diseases
- has cardiovascular benefits
- is excellent for brain health, preventing, or at least delaying, dementias
- decreases visceral fat
- adjusts our hunger and satiety hormones
- increases HGH-Human Growth Hormone in the body
- can "reset" the gut microbiome
- increases the healing natural body process of autophagy
- weight loss, if weight loss is indicated

*Health benefit descriptions and specific scientific research citations available in *Fast. Feast. Repeat.* by Gin Stephens.

Hundreds of thousands of people worldwide practice IF for weight management and overall health. It is not a quick weight-loss method, but by managing your food in a period of time each day, weight loss happens at a slow, healthy rate. As much as we all want to lose weight, overall health and wellness are the ultimate goals.

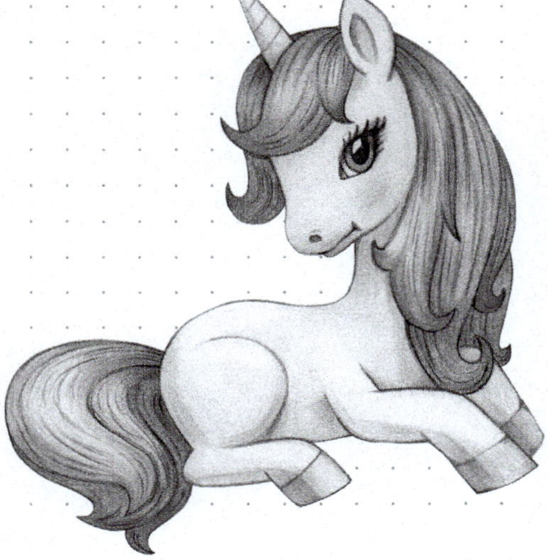

# *The HOW of Intermittent Fasting - AKA, Keep it Simple

Welcome to those who are new to the concept of IF. You are going to be amazed how practicing IF is going to help you on the path to accomplishing the health and weight-loss goals that you have set for yourself. This food management tool, combined with the five wellness habits that you will learn through completing this workbook, is going to change your life!

Because IF is the foundation of this book, I am going to save you lots of research time by directing you to the resources you need to quickly get up to speed , and begin your own IF experience. My own journey was informed by many books, all detailed in the resources section, but the most crucial are two by Gin Stephens: *Delay, Don't Deny* and *Fast. Feast. Repeat.*

To readers who are already practitioners of IF, congratulations! You already know what powerful benefits this practice offers. Now, you are ready to incorporate the five wellness habits, which, combined with your IF practice, will enable you to become the best version of you, for the rest of your life; a healthy, happy and content individual!

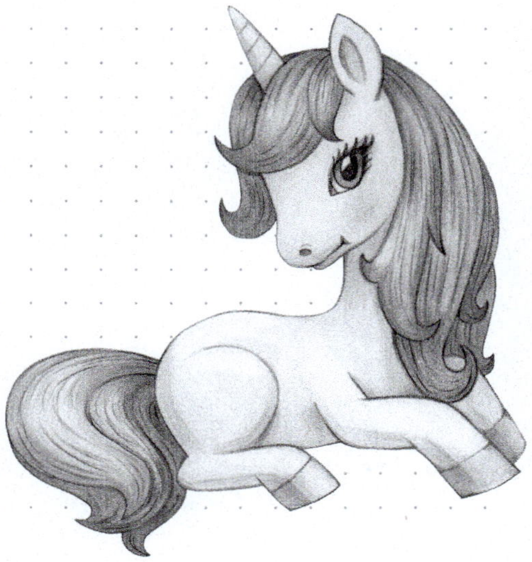

# *The CLEAN Fast

This concept is so foundational to IF, that it bears reviewing. The magic is in the clean fast! And make no mistake, there is no such thing as a "dirty fast." Either you are clean fasting, or you are not fasting.

The following are approved clean fast beverages:

Black coffee. Yes, black coffee really does mean just black coffee. No cream, sugar, sweeteners, heavy whipping cream, nothing. Period.

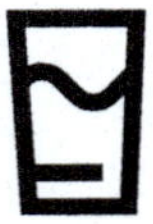

Plain water, and unflavored sparkling or mineral water. Nothing added, no lemon or other fruit or flavors, no sweeteners, nothing. Period.

Green or black tea – plain, unsweetened tea. No lemon, honey, sugar, sweeteners, or other flavors of any kind, nothing. Period.

Refer to the Clean Fast chart in Part 3: Fast with Paige "PLUS"

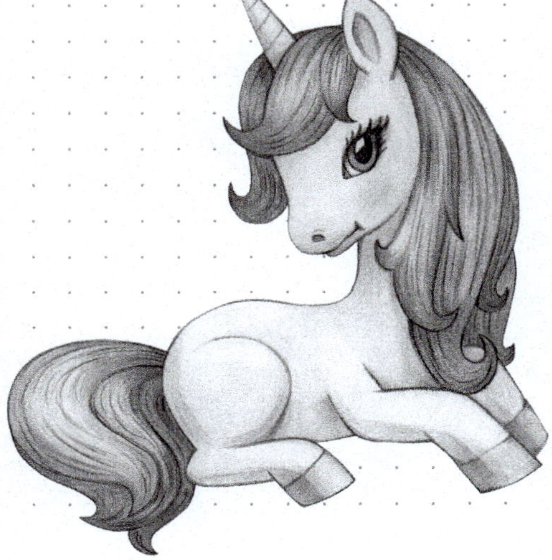

# *What is a "Window"?

Your daily eating "window" is such an important concept that it bears reviewing.

Every day you cycle between periods of clean fasting and a specific time each day when you eat.

This time during which you eat is called your eating "window." The length of time of your window is your choice and depends on your goals. For specific questions, refer to *Delay, Don't Deny* or *Fast. Feast. Repeat.* by Gin Stephens.

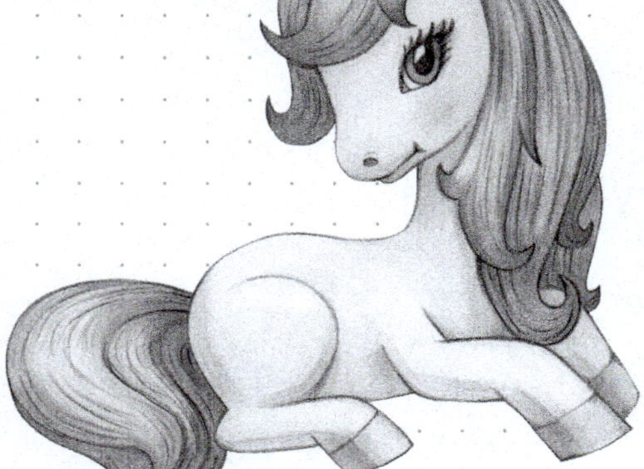

# *Empowerment: YOU Are in Charge at All Times!

*em*pow*er*ment*

- the process of becoming stronger and more confident, especially in controlling one's life and claiming one's rights.

A sense of empowerment was a missing piece during all my years of yo-yo dieting, the weight roller coaster that I just couldn't get off of, the search for "the answer" to what was going to finally "'fix"' me.

I got the message early in life that if you want to lose weight, you must go somewhere for help. You had to join gyms and weight-loss programs, take prescription medications, follow strict diet regimens with charts of good and bad foods, dictating exactly what to do and when to do it. If you couldn't follow the program, boy, were you in trouble! You were a failure, reduced to quitting and trying the next program that came along, hoping beyond hope that this program would be THE one.

I'm here to share the truth with you. You are not broken. You do not need to be fixed. What you DO need is to take back your sense of empowerment. You have the ability, the intelligence, the strength, and the wisdom to make good decisions for yourself about your health and wellness. You are wiser than you realize. No one knows you better than you know yourself. You oversee your life, and no one else. Reclaim your power! Personally, I never knew I had this power within myself all along.

You have the power to decide what foods to eat, and what foods work for your body. It takes practice, mindfulness, and paying attention to what your body is telling you. You'll learn, and the more you practice, the better you will get.

You have the power to become an intuitive eater. When I read that intermittent fasters gradually crave healthier foods and naturally make wiser food choices than in the past, I was skeptical. "They don't know me!" I thought. I'm never going to crave vegetables, and if left to my own devices (meaning if there wasn't a "diet" that I was following to make me make good choices), I'd choose ice cream over fruit every time!

I'd heard of the concept of intuitive eating, but to me, that was the "unicorn" of the weight-loss world. Either I was on a diet and following the rules, or I was NOT on a diet, making every horrible food choice you can imagine. I couldn't trust myself to be an intuitive eater! But when I empowered myself to begin IF, I unwittingly empowered myself to truly become an intuitive eater. And it can happen for you, too!

There are no food lists when you practice IF, no good foods or bad foods. There are foods that you enjoy and make you feel great when you eat them. There are taste treats that you enjoy choosing occasionally. And always, you're in charge and what you eat is your decision. You're empowered to make good choices for you and your body.

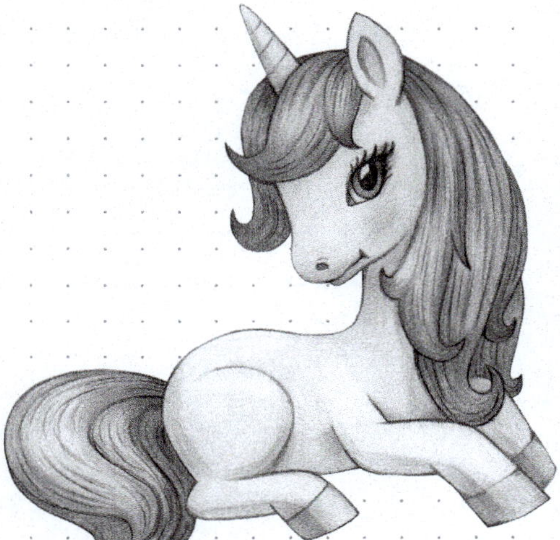

# *Trust the Process to Regain Trust in Yourself

Quite honestly, becoming empowered to make decisions for myself was scary. Years of failed diet history left me believing I couldn't make good decisions on my own. Within the framework of a diet, I had a track record of making good choices. I lost weight following many different diets, so I knew I was capable of making wise choices.

But, these good decisions were guided by outside forces like diet programs. Every diet I ever tried, I eventually quit. Once I quit the diet, I went immediately back to my terrible eating habits. I stopped making good decisions for myself with my food choices. Either I was dieting, or I was gaining.

Because of my history, I was fearful.

That fear, as well as a lack of trust in myself, were major stumbling blocks in becoming empowered. They blocked my ability to successfully take charge of my health, lose weight, and keep it off.

For me, the solution to overcoming my fear and my lack of trust in myself, came from a suggestion in Gin Stephens' *Delay, Don't Deny*: trust the process.

Trust the process? What exactly did that mean? I excel when I have details and things are clear to me, and it took me awhile to figure out what the phrase "trust the process" really meant. Broken down, to trust the process of IF, to be committed to the process, looks like this:

- Keep a clean fast every single day, no matter how long or how short the fast.
- Honor both your clean fast and your eating window, daily.
- When your window is closed, it is closed. Period.
- Decide how many hours you want to fast, and then fast that number of hours, every single day, without fail.
- Take it one day at a time. Keep the process simple. Fast, feast, repeat!

And that is what I did. I didn't think about the fact that I'd never been able to trust myself before. I couldn't handle thinking about that. I just followed the steps above, and I trusted the process of intermittent fasting. I kept it simple: fasted and then feasted daily. Over time, I developed a new track record. I was making good choices with increasing ease, and this gave me confidence. I became empowered, and by trusting the process, I proved that I could trust myself, after all!

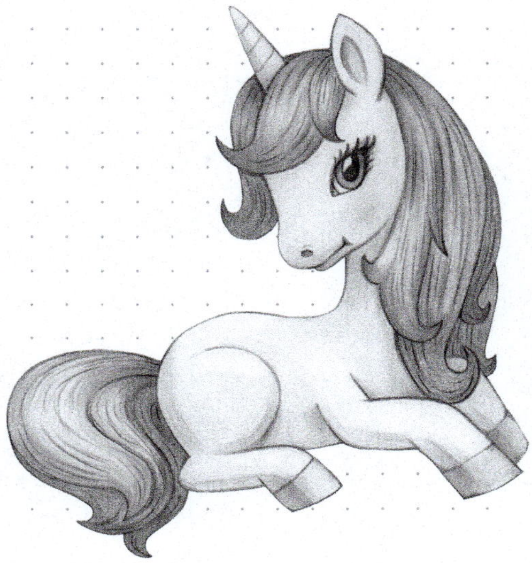

# *Breaking Through Limiting Beliefs

What are limiting beliefs? They are any belief or thought that keeps you from believing that you can be successful in taking charge or your health and life.

Have you ever told yourself any of the following?

- I can't lose weight on my own.
- I'll never be able to lose weight and keep it off.
- I'm a failure. I have failed at every weight loss attempt I've ever made.
- I am going to be this way forever. It is just the way it is.
- It is genetics. I can't control it; how can I change my genes?
- I have no choice except to be overweight forever.
- I might as well eat whatever I want, since I am always going to be this way.
- Intermittent fasting is not going to work. I am just going to get even fatter with no rules or food lists to help me know what to eat.
- I'm never going to be a healthy weight. It just is not in the cards for me.
- I have to count calories, track macros, or weigh my food to lose weight. That is the only way it's going to happen.
- No one will ever love me because I am fat.
- I might as well quit trying;, I just cannot lose weight.
- If I cannot be perfect in my food choices, if I make a mistake, I have to start over next Monday...next month...next year.
- I'm not good enough.
- I must be skinny before I can be in a relationship.
- I can't practice intermittent fasting. I could never go that long without food!
- I could NEVER (fill in the blank)!

Part of the responsibility of being empowered to take charge of your life is to be honest with yourself. We always believe what we tell ourselves. Each of these limiting beliefs are lies that we tell ourselves out of negative emotion. It may be what we feel, but it is not the truth!

PART TWO

# Fast with Paige PRACTICES - Wellness Habits

As you first become aware of the five Wellness Habits, then learn to practice and incorporate them into your life, you'll learn how to truly be honest with yourself. Freedom from limiting beliefs allows you to grow; to become the best version of you; to be happy, healthy, and content!

Along with the foundational practice of IF, there are five things to incorporate into your daily life in order to change your mindset and lifestyle from those of an unhealthy, out-of-control person, to someone empowered to take charge of their life, health, and wellness. You'll adopt the identity of someone capable of losing weight and keeping it off long-term.

The five Wellness Habits are:

1. Self-Love & and Self-Acceptance
2. Empowered Thinking
3. Self-Honoring Choices
4. Positive Mindset
5. Joyful Movement

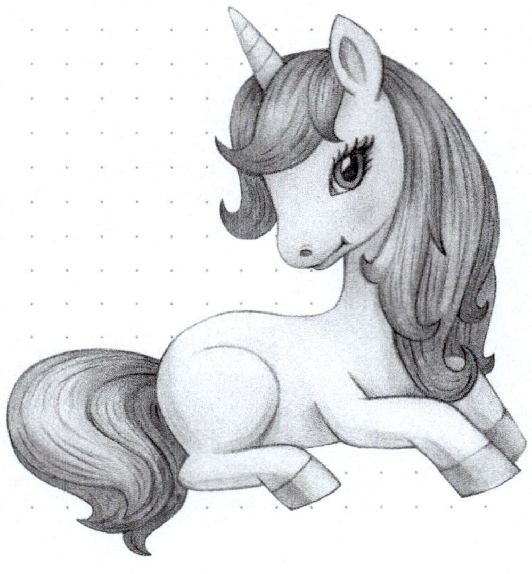

# *The Five-Week Guide to Set You Up for Success

For the next five weeks, you will be introduced to a new wellness habit each week. You will learn about that habit, amplifying your awareness of each.

The key to making permanent shifts in your mindset and lifestyle is to implement the cycle of improvement:

1. Awareness – identify what you need to improve.

2. Deliberate practice – focus your conscious effort on the specific area you want to improve.

3. Habit – with consistent, intentional practice, the habit becomes an automatic action.

Each week, you'll have the opportunity to identify actions to take in order to build the identified wellness habit, choose activities to assist you in practicing those actions, and incorporate the habits into your life.

Each week is an introduction, a. A roadmap for you to continue to refine and make changes as needed. At the end of the five weeks, you'll have an introduction to each of the wellness habits, and will be ready to continue on your path to mindset and lifestyle change. In short, you will be ready to fly!

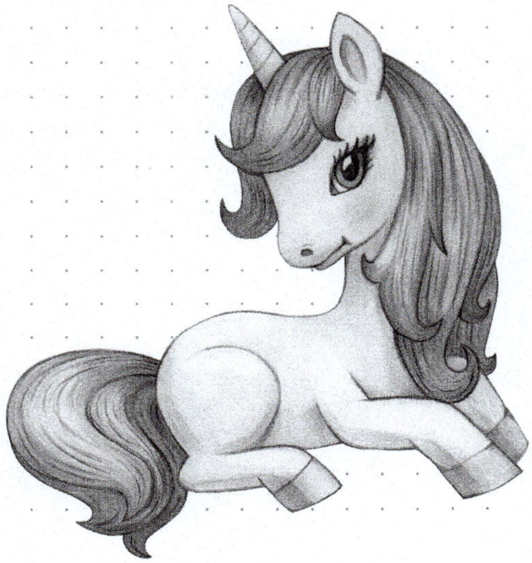

# WEEK 1 FOCUS:
# Self-Love & Self-Acceptance

What does it mean to love yourself? Doesn't everyone automatically love themselves? If asked, most people would say, "Of course, I love myself!" What would YOU say, and do your actions reflect true self-love?

For too many years, my actions certainly did not reflect love for myself. I ate terribly unhealthy foods daily. I didn't get enough sleep. I got very little healthy movement; in fact, I was a couch potato. I did not purchase fun, cute clothes that made me feel confident. I thought I had to wait until I finally lost the weight to dress fashionably. If I received a gift of lovely perfume, I'd put it away for a special occasion. What was I waiting for? Sadly, I did not recognize that life itself is a special occasion and I deserve to be nurtured. Self-acceptance was clearly not in my vocabulary, but it is now.

You deserve to feel amazing and confident. Loving yourself is recognizing that you're an amazing person right now, just as you are. Your worth is not determined by your size. That thought reflects a limiting belief. You are a complex, interesting, vibrant person with countless positive attributes and people who love you. Today. No matter your size.

One vital expression of self-love is shown in the way you talk to yourself. For many years, my self-talk was harsh, impatient, hateful, critical, depressing, and lacking compassion for myself. I failed to give myself grace. How can you feel positivity and love toward yourself when you speak in a way you would never speak to anyone else?

Self-care is too often ignored, especially by busy women. We are caretakers for our families. We have jobs, commitments, PTA meetings, church services, business meetings, and often are also caretakers for our aging parents. In our stressful, busy lives, who has time for a bubble bath?

Any activity that nurtures and refuels you is a self-care activity. These activities will differ from person to person. It's critical to incorporate self-care into your day. When your own tank is filled up, you can serve others better. You cannot care for others in a loving way if you are exhausted, depleted, and inevitably feeling resentful. Taking care of yourself is not selfish; it must be a top priority for your mental, emotional, and physical wellbeing. When you are nourished, you can give from a place of love and overflow.Consistent, quality self-care has positive ripple effects on both your personal and professional success, and your loved ones will reap the benefits.

*Dad goes to the gym: "I am being so healthy!"*
*Mom goes to the gym: "I am being so selfish!"*

Sound familiar? Give yourself permission to engage in self-care activities, to have a fulfilling life and experience optimal health. Health is not just the absence of disease, but a state of complete physical, mental, and emotional wellbeing.

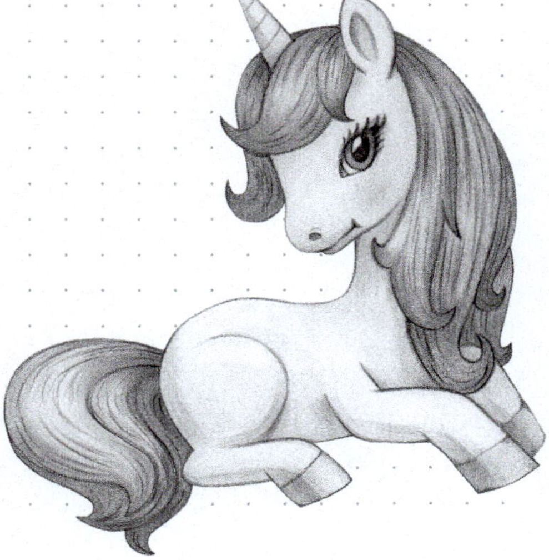

Empowerment comes into play in self-care. Take ownership of your needs. Let your loved ones know what you need, along with identifying what they need.

The expected outcome of empowering yourself to love and accept yourself fully is experiencing optimal health and happiness.

## **Activity Selections & Scheduling*

Select activities to reinforce the new wellness habit and schedule them into your week. Be thoughtful and intentional as you participate in them. The more effort and thought you put into the activities, the more you will benefit from them.

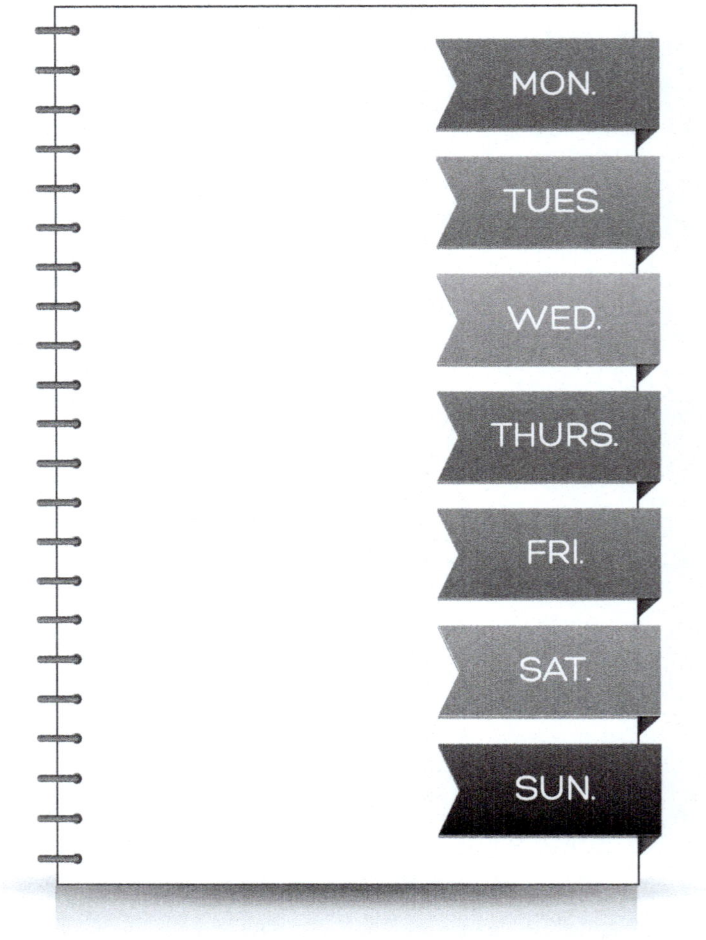


## *Activity Selection*

WRITE A LOVE LETTER TO YOURSELF

In your letter, first establish that you are an incredible person, right now, just as you are. Explain all the reasons that you are wonderful. Be specific and list the positive qualities that make you – YOU!

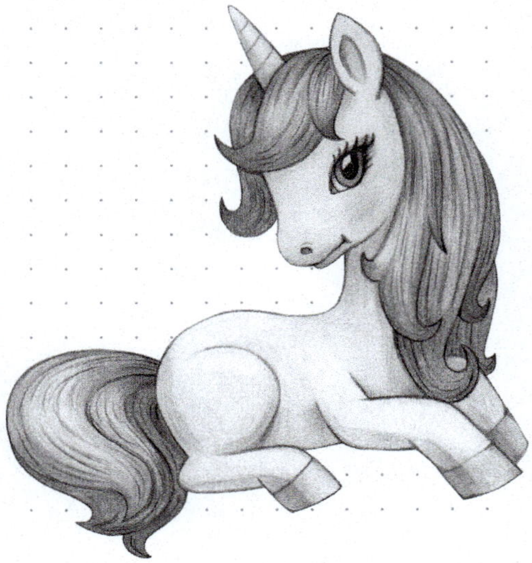

Brainstorm and describe some ways that you can show yourself more self-love. What activities can you incorporate into your life that will fulfill you emotionally, physically, and mentally? How will you find the time to practice them? In your letter, outline activities that can be done very quickly, some that can be accomplished with a bit of advanced planning, and some that will require some serious "me" time.

And finally, in your letter, outline how you will let your family and loved ones know what you need. They are not mind readers, and it's important to make your needs known.

## *Activity Selection*

### CONCEPT MAPPING

A concept map is a graphical representation of information and knowledge. They are helpful to understand how two concepts can be related and might affect each other.

Steps:

1. Consider the following question: "Is there a relationship between self-love and setting healthy boundaries?"
2. Define each of the two concepts introduced in the statement above.
3. Draw a concept map detailing the relationship between the two concepts using shapes like squares and circles, connecting lines, labeled arrows, etc.
4. Elaborate on the relational links that you identify.
5. Are these concepts more similar or different?
6. Write an explanation of how they relate to each other in the form of a conclusion statement.

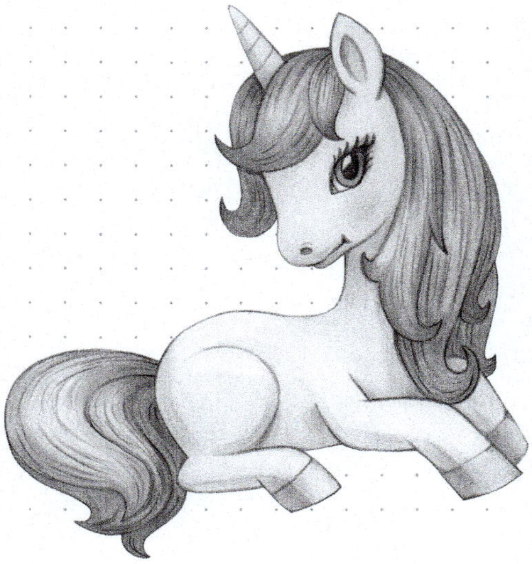

## *Activity Selection*

HALT THE TALK!

If negative self-talk is an issue for you, you are going to monitor your self-talk very closely. Every single time you catch yourself engaging in self-talk that is punitive, mean, impatient, negative, critical, or just plain hateful, follow these steps. Every. Single. Time. This takes intentional practice, persistence, and consistency. Keep doing this, and over time, you'll find your negative self-talk has become positive, loving, kind, and gentle.

1. When you realize you are engaging in negative self-talk, immediately say STOP! to yourself.
2. Think of a person that you love with all your heart: a parent, sibling, child, or friend.
3. Think of that person and imagine that they are in your same exact situation.
4. What would you say to this person in this same circumstance?
5. Inevitably, it would be something kind, loving, and above all – truthful!! (Note: be objective and honest here. For example, was it really your friend's fault that her boss yelled at her because she was stupid? Of course not! Her boss likely yelled at her because of being stressed out or in a bad mood. She is a great employee.)
6. Now, say that exact thing to YOURSELF!
7. This takes lots of practice to become a habit!! But, the more you do it, the more you find that instead of speaking badly to yourself, you will automatically say to yourself what you would say to that person that you love.
8. Over time, you will become your own best friend! Speak to yourself, always, like you would your best friend or that loved one.

## **Reflection and Application*

EXIT SLIP

Jot down what you learned about the habit of self-love & and self-acceptance.

Discuss how incorporating self-love & and self-acceptance into your life will help you live a healthy lifestyle moving forward. How will doing so help you make a mindset shift?

List at least 5 five actions that you will incorporate into your schedule on a regular basis to help self-love & and self-acceptance become an automatic wellness habit in your life.

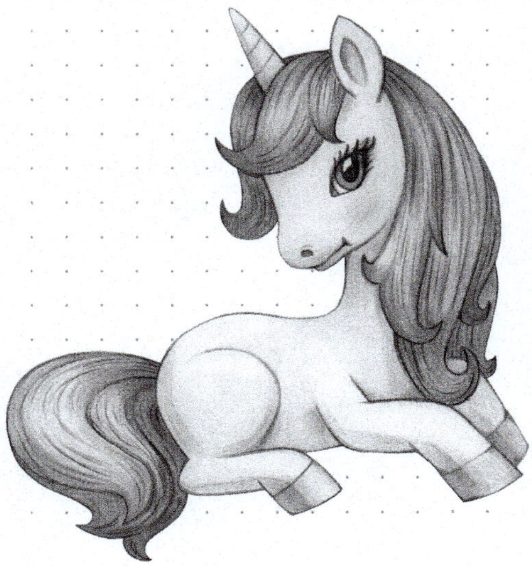

# WEEK 2 FOCUS:
# Empowered Thinking

Do any of these thoughts feel familiar to you?

- I want weight loss results NOW!
- If I do not lose lots of weight every week, I'm a failure and might as well quit.
- I must be perfect on a diet, or I might as well quit.
- If I eat good food, I'm a good person, and when I eat bad food, I'm a bad person.
- I have blown it for today, I'll just start over next Monday...or next month...or next year.
- I must follow a diet to be able to lose weight.
- Either I am all on a diet or I'm all off.
- Exercise is a necessary evil.
- Look at how fast my friend is losing. It is not fair, I am working harder than she is!

Collectively, this type of disordered, unhealthy thinking is called "diet brain". Diet brain is the kind of thinking that we develop over time with unsuccessful diets we try. The more diet failures we experience, the more ingrained these types of thoughts become. These had been my thoughts for so many years, that I did not even realize they weren't normal thoughts. I did not realize that they weren't true. How does one know their thinking is disordered when it is how they have been thinking as long as they can remember? Diet brain keeps us stuck, doomed to keep repeating the same behaviors while hoping for a different outcome. Diet brain is made up of limiting beliefs.

The key to eliminating these limiting beliefs is to first become aware that they are disordered, unhealthy, and untrue. To realize that you are telling yourself things that are not the truth.

Replacing diet brain thoughts is a matter of recognizing them as they happen, and replacing them with healthy, truthful thoughts.

You can empower yourself to redirect your thoughts, and to continue practicing doing this, until you have replaced these limiting beliefs with truthful, healthy thoughts. As with your food choices, you are in control of your thoughts and beliefs.

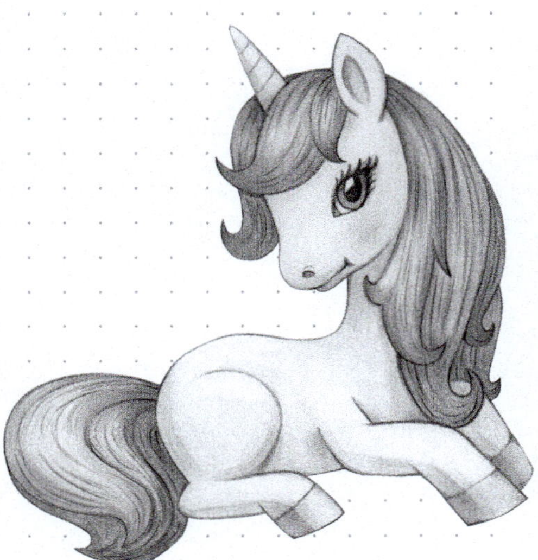

What does healthy thinking look like? Here are some examples:

- Time is my friend.; I know I did not gain this weight overnight, and I know that slow, steady weight loss is the healthiest way to lose weight.
- I make conscious choices about what I am going to eat. I own my choices, enjoy whatever I have decided to eat, and move on.
- Some foods serve my body well and make me feel great.! Other foods are wonderful to enjoy occasionally for the pure delight of it.
- I eat food for energy, nutrition, to live, to feel well and for life enjoyment. Food is not good or bad.
- I practice IF every day; I don't diet. I eat food that I want, food that makes me feel great, and that food I enjoy.
- I am empowered to make the best food choices for my body.
- The exercise that I choose to engage in is pleasurable, makes me feel great both mentally and physically, adds years to my life, and helps prevent many lifestyle-related diseases.
- The number on the scale is merely a data point and not the best indicator of success; non-scale victories are THE best and most exciting way to measure progress.
- By practicing IF, I am just living my life, honoring my daily fast and eating window while eating what I want, and moving on.

Continue to practice replacing unhealthy, false, negative thoughts with healthy thoughts. The more you practice, the sooner healthy thinking will become an automatic habit, which is the expected outcome of practicing this wellness habit.

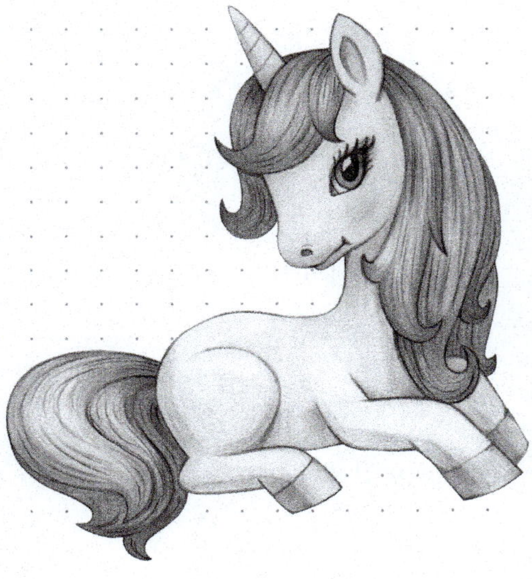

## **Activity Selections & and Scheduling*

Select activities to reinforce the new wellness habit and schedule them into your week. Be thoughtful and intentional as you participate in them. The more effort and thought you put into the activities, the more you will benefit from them.

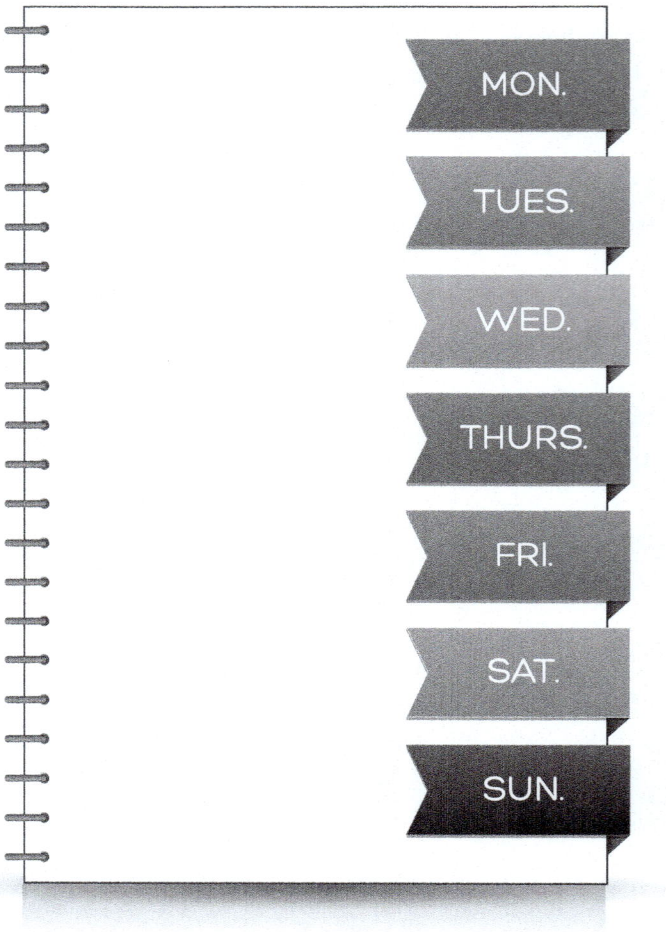


## *Activity Selection*

MYSTERY QUOTE

- Read the quote below. Figure out the point of view of the person who is being quoted.
- Write a justification of why you believe that this is their point of view. Do you agree with it? Explain why or why not.
- Does this relate to your current situation? How so?
- Identify any actions that you would like to take as this relates to your situation.

**"Yesterday is heavy; let it go."**

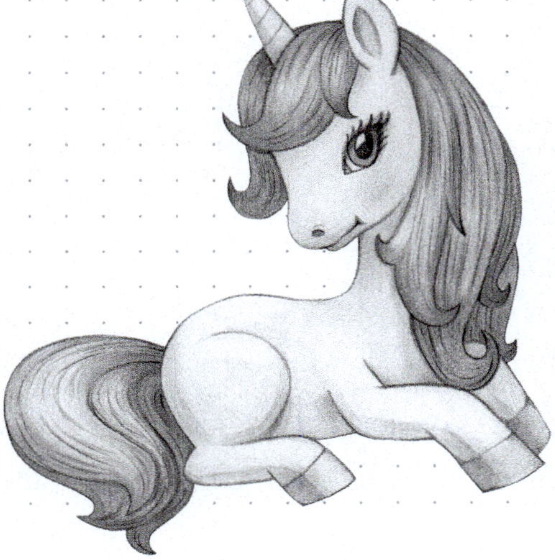

## *Activity Selection*

LENGTHEN THE LIST

Brainstorm a list of every non-scale victory that you have had to date. Think of every improvement, victory, win, and happy occurrence that have come about due to living an IF lifestyle. Keep this list going! Every single non-scale victory you experience, no matter how small, add it to the list. Non-scale victories are great measures of success, and nothing motivates like success. Notice and celebrate your non-scale victories every day and read through this list any time you need a boost or encouragement.

## *Activity Selection*

PRO/CON GRID

Eliminating negative thinking and limiting beliefs is work that is necessary is work that is necessary to do to achieve long-term health and weight-loss goals.

Create a grid listing the pros and cons, or the negatives and positives, associated with the work of eliminating limiting beliefs. List at least 5 five examples for each category.

## *Activity Selection*

REAL-TIME REACTIONS

Write your answers to the following questions:

1. How did reading the list of diet-brain thinking make you feel? Explain why.
2. Do you have any diet-brain type of thoughts that weren't listed? What are they?
3. How did reading the list of healthy thoughts make you feel? Explain why.
4. Have you had any healthy thoughts regarding food choices and IF that weren't listed? What are they?
5. What will your life look like if you constantly think healthy, truthful thoughts?

## **Reflection and Application*

EXIT SLIP

Jot down what you learned about the wellness habit of healthy thinking.

Discuss how incorporating healthy thinking into your life will help you live a healthy lifestyle moving forward. How will doing so help you make a mindset shift?

List at least 5 five actions that you will incorporate into your schedule on a regular basis to help healthy thinking become an automatic wellness habit in your life.

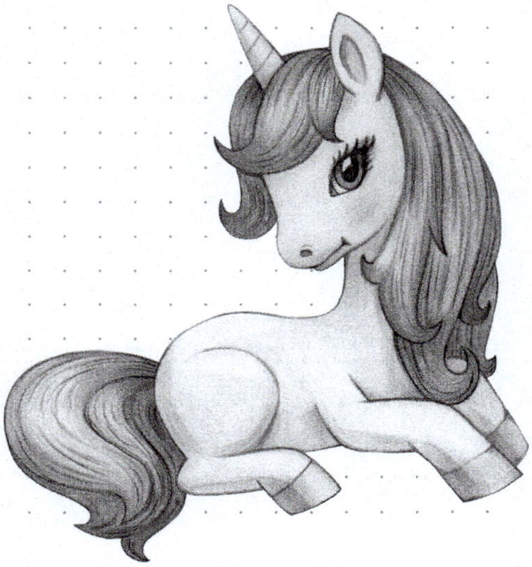

# WEEK 3 FOCUS:
# Self-Honoring Choices

Identifying healthy habits, practicing them daily, and gaining mastery so that they become automatic is a form of "health insurance". Our habits drive our lives and determine our lifestyles. In order to make a lifestyle shift from that of an unhealthy or obese person to the lifestyle of an active, healthy, happy person, you must eliminate unhealthy habits and replace them with healthy ones.

During my work with a therapist, we determined that I did not have an eating disorder or food addiction; I had a complete lack of empowerment or control over my own life. I suffered from disordered thinking, or the "diet-brain" thoughts that I'd held since I was a teen. And just as damaging were my unhealthy habits controlling my life and my poor health, and literally causing me to be morbidly obese. These habits included:

- I seldom cooked or ate at home.
- On most days I ate out, all three meals.
- Most of these restaurant meals were fast food.
- I ate a large meal 3X/day and was eating much more food than my body needed.
- I never got anywhere near the recommended 7-8 hours of sleep each night.
- My diet was heavy in processed foods and sweets.
- I only ate fruits and vegetables during those brief times when I was "on a diet".

I understood that during those times that I was trying to follow a diet, I ate much healthier and made better choices. But, the diets never lasted more than a matter of months, at which time I would quit and continue my downward spiral.

I never made the connection that the way I ate was due to habits. It was just the way I ate. I felt no sense of control over the way I ate. Just like being morbidly obese, it just seemed like the way it was, and I felt powerless to change anything.

What do healthy habits look like? They can range from surrounding yourself with other like-minded people who are on the same health and weight-loss path as you, to getting adequate sleep, or to engaging in meaningful self-care.

How do you begin to cultivate healthy habits? For me, it started with practicing intermittent fasting. Just by doing that, I was forced to stop a lot of my bad habits. I had to choose. Continue these horrible habits, or begin my IF lifestyle.

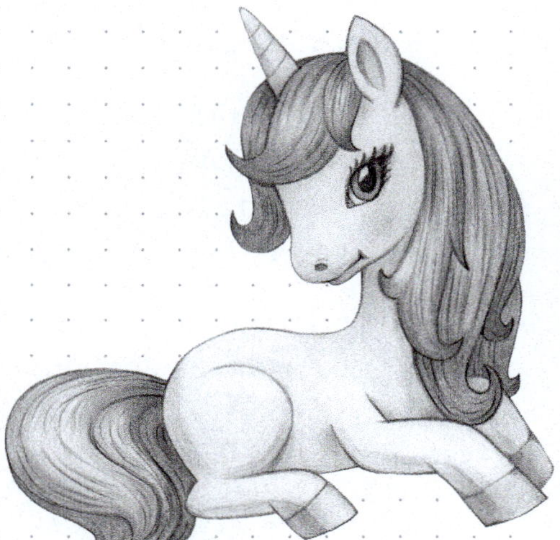

I chose IF and never looked back. I did not even realize it at the time, but the first healthy habit I started was to practice a clean fast every day. And to eat my food in a window every day.

If you want to master a habit, the key is to identify the habit you wish to start and then take that action every day. Every habit begins with repetition. Not only is it common sense, it is research based; repetition causes change. Some helpful tips when beginning a healthy habit include:

- Make it as easy as possible. Motivation and willpower are great, but fickle. Successful people set themselves up for success by making their behavior changes as easy as they can.
- Control your environment. If you don't buy your trigger foods at the grocery store, you won't eat them. It is that simple.
- Do not confuse your goal with your habit. You need healthy habits to reach your goal. Your goal may be to run a marathon, but your initial important first step/habit is to put on your running shoes every day.
- Consistency is crucial in beginning and cultivating a new habit.
- Think positive thoughts to encourage your habits. Instead of thinking "I have to walk before work this morning," think "I'm happy I'm able to walk before work today!" Negative emotions pull you back into bad habits, like hitting the snooze and ditching your morning walk.
- Do not expect to be 100% perfect; progress, not perfection, is the goal.
- Make the new habit enjoyable. If you enjoy checking boxes off a to-do list, create a chart and mark off every day you practice the new habit. If you love to listen to music or podcasts, always listen to them while you walk.
- Be very mindful, and celebrate each day when you practice that new habit. Feeling immediate success helps us stick with new habits.
- Keep a log or a running list of your healthy new habits, and add to it each day. Nothing is as motivating as success. Make your success visible in some way.
- Fall in love with the healthy habit of daily fasting and eating within your window. If you genuinely enjoy the process on a daily basis, you can focus on that and be happy now. No more "waiting till I get to goal" or "waiting until I finally lose the weight" to be happy. Be happy every day because you are really enjoying the process of IF.
- Take pride and joy when you begin to practice the habit without even thinking about it. The goal is for the action to become automatic and effortless.

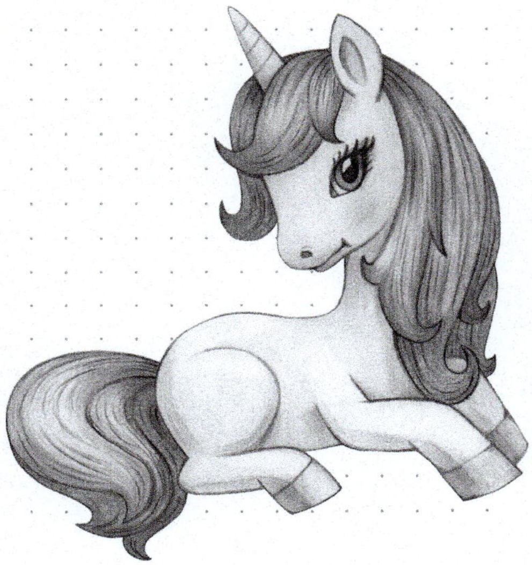

Motivation may be what gets you started, but habit is what keeps you going. Your focus should be on the daily actions you take, and the habits you create, not the results you are seeking. If you focus on results, you'll never change. If you focus on change, you will get results! Therefore, focusing on the daily practice of IF, rather than focusing on what the scale says every day, helps you achieve success.

Continue to identify more healthy habits to incorporate into your day as your healthy habits become automatic. As I moved further along with my IF practice, I realized I wasn't really focusing on my fasts anymore. I just did them automatically, which freed up mental space to begin incorporating other healthy habits. One secret to getting results that last, the very thing we are seeking, is to never stop improving, one healthy habit at a time.

One month from now, are you going to have a month's worth of progress under your belt, or are you going to have a month's worth of excuses why you do not? As always, the choice is yours.

## **Activity Selections & and Scheduling*

Select activities to reinforce the new wellness habit and schedule them into your week. Be thoughtful and intentional as you participate in them. The more effort and thought you put into the activities, the more you will benefit from them.

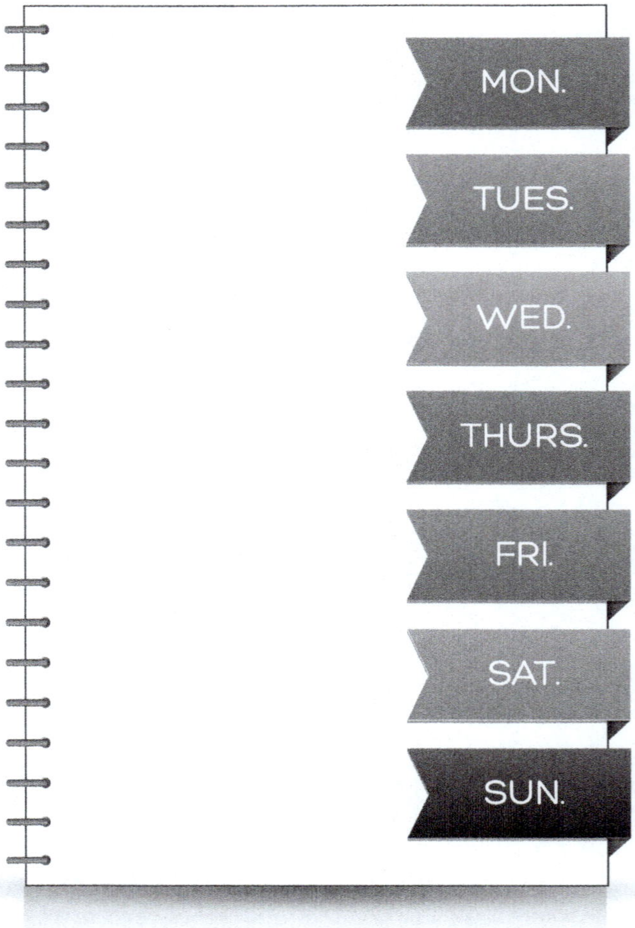

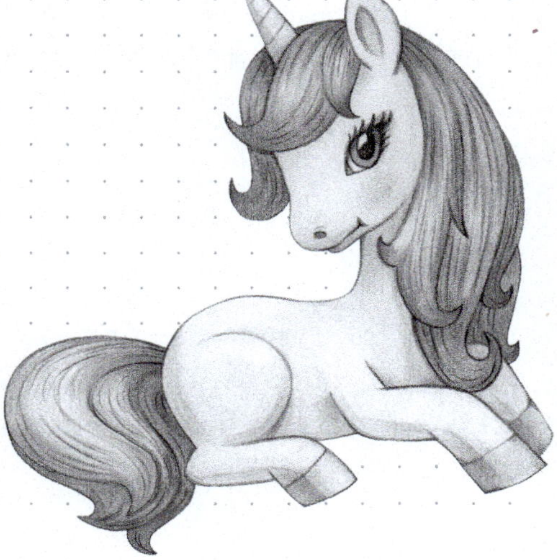

## *Activity Selection*

TRIPLE PLAY

Create a list of unhealthy habits that you can identify in your current daily or weekly routine. Beside each, detail how it is a stumbling block to reaching your health, weight loss and wellness goals.

Now create a second list, this one of healthy habits that you currently practice. Remember the obvious ones, like brushing and flossing your teeth each day, and showering regularly. Show how each habit helps you in achieving health, weight loss and wellness goals.

Finally, create a list of healthy habits that you would like to incorporate into your life. Explain how each of these is going to assist you in attaining your health, weight loss and wellness goals.

## *Activity Selection*

SKETCH-NOTING

Sketch a picture that represents what you have learned about unhealthy habits and healthy habits. By doing so, you will be creating a way to visualize your understanding. Make your sketch as detailed as possible.

After you complete the sketch, imagine that you are presenting the sketch to classmates. Write at least two paragraphs about what you would say to explain your sketch.

## *Activity Selection*

VENN DIAGRAM

Create a Venn Diagram. Label one circle Unhealthy Habits. Label the other circle Healthy Habits. The intersection will contain current habits (both healthy and unhealthy). Upon completion, create an action plan for yourself based on the results of your Venn Diagramdiagram. What unhealthy habits do you want to extinguish? What healthy habits do you want to start? Are there any current habits you will continue?

## *Activity Selection*

REFLECT OUT LOUD!

Write down four reflections from your learning on healthy habits. Choose someone to share these reflections with. It can be a spouse, friend, other family member, or online friend. Share how you plan to incorporate this information into your life moving forward.

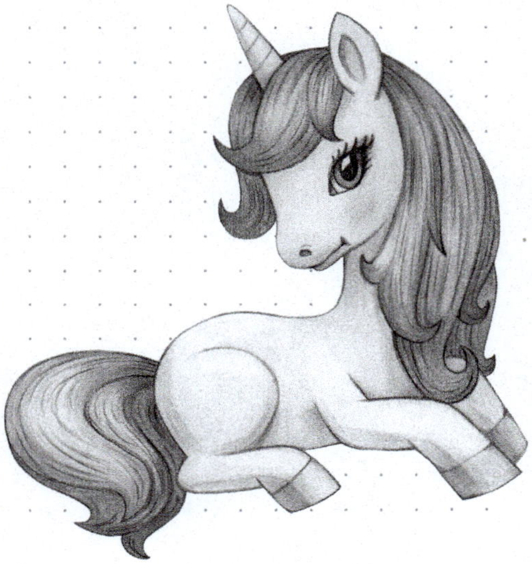

## **Reflection and Application*

EXIT SLIP

Jot down what you learned about the wellness habit of healthy habits.

Discuss how incorporating healthy habits into your life will help you live a healthy lifestyle moving forward. How will doing so help you make a mindset shift?

List at least 5 five actions that you will incorporate into your schedule on a regular basis to help healthy habits become an automatic wellness habit in your life.

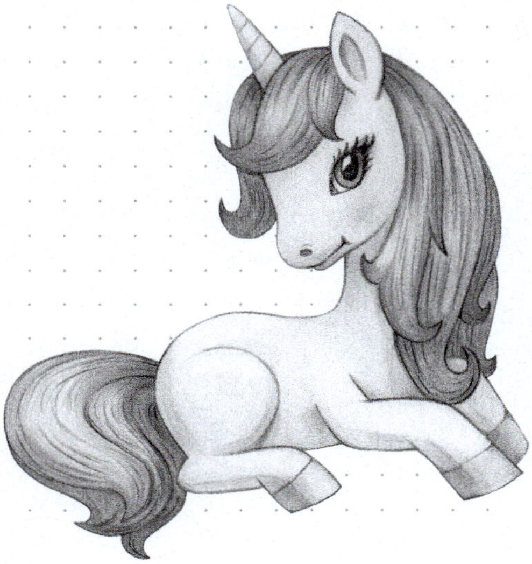

# WEEK 4 FOCUS:
# Positive Mindset

We believe what we tell ourselves. I'm sure you've heard the old adage, "Whether you think you can, or you think you can't, you're right."

It's not an accident that a positive mindset is identified as a wellness habit. The truth is, being positive is a habit. Looking for the positives in a situation is an intentional act. Thinking positive thoughts is a mindful activity. No one is automatically positive all the time, but we all can cultivate this habit, and be a person who's automatically positive most of the time.

Nobody disputes that a positive mindset is a crucial shift to achieving long-term health and weight-loss goals. I guarantee you that each time I "fell off the diet wagon" and sank into the familiar downward spiral of unhealthy choices and weight regain: my thoughts were incredibly negative.

Bad days happen, too, right? Who can be positive all the time? We can all recognize that not every day is a great day, but we can also find some good in every day, even when we must look a little harder. Cultivating a positive mindset is not to bury your head in the sand. If you look for positive things, you can always find them, even on the difficult days.

You can choose the kind of day you're going to have before you even get out of bed in the morning. You consciously choose your attitude, which drives whether you have a good day or a bad day. And if yesterday wasn't such a great day? Don't ruin a good today by choosing to dwell on yesterday. Let it go! The more you practice, the more automatic these thoughts become.

A positive mindset is extremely helpful when making food choices in your window. Get into the habit of asking, "Does this choice support my goals?" Our weight-loss goals support our overarching goals of enjoying great health, overall wellness, and a feeling of contentment.

A positive mindset also helps with one of the most challenging aspects of weight loss: being patient. Understanding that we didn't become obese and unhealthy overnight, we need to accept that reversing these conditions takes time and patience. We won't reach our ultimate weight-loss goal overnight, but if we give up, it won't happen at all. Thinking this way gives us the ability to appreciate that a little progress each day adds up to big results. While the magic is the clean fast, patience is the "special sauce" that allows the magic to happen.

This mindset is key in realizing that our non-scale victories (NSVs) are critical to our motivation and day-to-day happiness. They are truly the good stuff in life, and by noticing and celebrating these accomplishments, small and large, we nourish ourselves and become able to practice that patience we used to find so difficult.

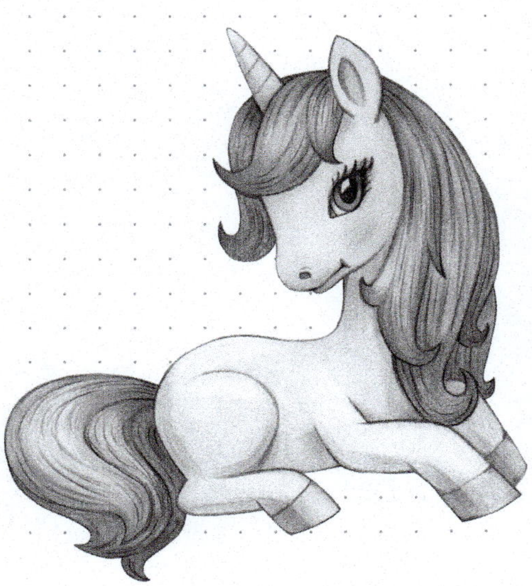

If you're like me, these ideas are not new to you. I'd heard them before, but never really understood the power of positive thinking before. I thought it was all pie in the sky 'woo- woo' stuff. I didn't comprehend that I could be empowered to choose my thoughts. I had a victim mentality, a negative mindset, and again, I just thought that was the way it was.

And finally, we all struggle; that is not going to change. Struggle is the intersection of success and failure. In the past, we've always chosen the path of failure by not choosing a positive mindset. Cultivating a positive mindset will help us choose the path to success.

In *Fast. Feast. Repeat.*, not only does Gin Stephens discuss the importance of mindset, she cites scientific research supporting the importance of having a positive mindset.

## **Activity Selections & and Scheduling*

Select from the provided activities to reinforce the wellness habit of positive mindset. Schedule these three activities into your week. Be specific about when you will do them. Also, be thoughtful and intentional as you participate in the activities. The more effort and thought you put into the activities, the more you will benefit from them.

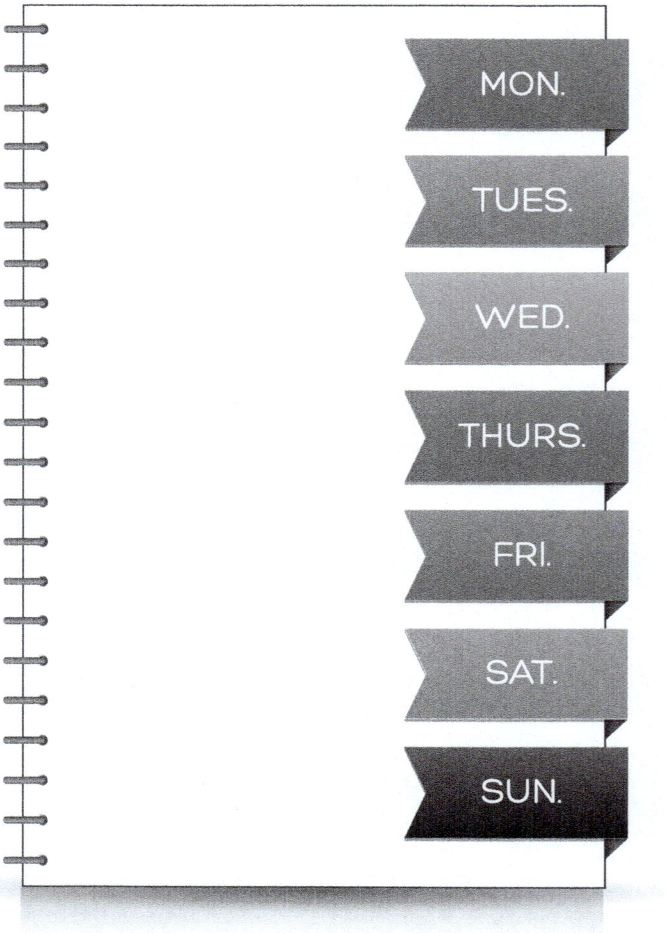

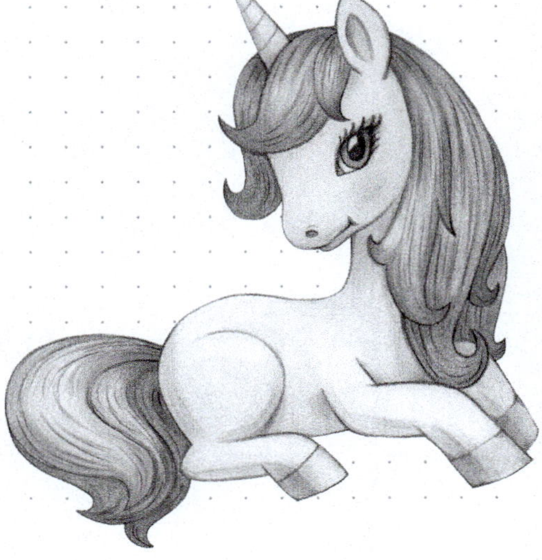

## *Activity Selection*

MYSTERY QUOTE

- Read the quote below. Figure out the point of view of the person being quoted. Write what you believe this point of view is.
- Write a justification of why you believe that this is their point of view. Do you agree with this point of view? Explain why or why not.
- Does this relate to you and your current situation? How so?
- Identify any actions that you need to take as this relates to your situation.

**"Good things come to those who BELIEVE, better things come to those who are PATIENT, and the best things come to those who DON'T GIVE UP!"**

## *Activity Selection*

CRYSTAL BALL

Imagine that you are gazing into a beautiful crystal ball. You can see yourself in the future. You are vibrant! You are the size you have always wanted to be, confident, happy, energetic, and content. You are the very picture of health.

Clearly, your mindset has shifted for your future self to be so healthy and happy. You close your eyes and imagine that you ARE that future self. How do you feel? What do you want to share with the current version of you? What hope can you offer? W, what would you tell that sad, unhealthy, defeated, frustrated version of yourself about what lies ahead because of living an IF lifestyle, and making the wellness habit changes you are learning about now?

Listen closely to the advice your future self shares, about all the mindset changes that are going to take place and help change your life!

Write these changes down in the form of a list. Choose a loved one and share these mindset changes.

## *Activity Selection*

ONE-MINUTE REFLECTIONS

Write the answer to each of these one-minute reflection questions. Be honest. Really consider each question. Be mindful of how the answers can benefit you, as you shift your mindset from negative to positive.

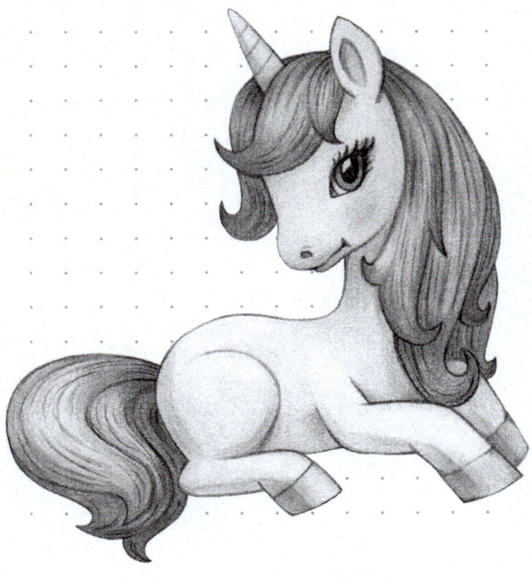

1. What was the most important thing you learned about your mindset?
2. Why was this the most important thing you learned?
3. What questions do you still have, and how do you intend to find the answers?
4. Why is a positive mindset considered a crucial wellness habit?
5. What point from this week's wellness habit work is the most meaningful to you?
6. What I enjoyed learning the most, that will really help me in my life, was __________.

## *Activity Selection*

### CASE STUDY ANALYSIS

Read the following case study:

Kelly grew up in a diet culture within her home.

Kelly's Dad dad was super thin, ate anything he wanted, and never gained a pound. He only ate when he was hungry; his whole family was thin.

Kelly's Mom mom alternated between being overweight, obese, or morbidly obese. Practically the whole side of her Mom's family fits into one of these categories. Kelly's Mom mom tried diet after diet, always losing some weight, until she quit and regained the weight, plus more. When a meeting style weight-loss organization opened in their city, Kelly's Mom mom was one of the original members, losing 100-plus pounds. Over the years, however, she regained the weight. She then tried other organized diet programs, losing over 100 pounds with two more of them, but ultimately regaining the weight each time.

Kelly had three sisters. All four were a healthy, normal weight. Kelly's sisters seemed to take after their Dad. But, Kelly loved food. She loved to eat, and she especially loved sweets!

Seeing this tendency in Kelly, her Mom mom became very fearful that Kelly was going down a familiar and difficult path. She did not want this for Kelly! In the best way she knew how, she tried to diminish this love of food in Kelly. She cautioned her about the food she was eating. She told her if she kept eating like she was, she was going to get fat. She limited Kelly's snacking. It broke her heart to think that Kelly might have the same weight problem that she did, and she tried desperately to stop it from happening.

Kelly did NOT like being told what she could and could not eat! Her solution was to sneak food into her room to eat when she wanted. Of course, she always got caught, and she got into trouble for that.

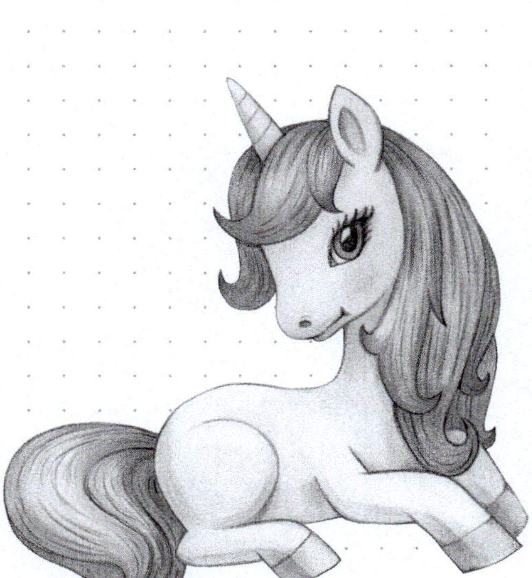

In her teens, Kelly was a bit overweight. Her Mom mom encouraged her to join the weekly in-person weight-loss program with her, so Kelly joined, and they attended weekly meetings together. Kelly's Mom mom encouraged her to reach her goal and become the organizations' FIRST first teenage meeting leader. That never happened.

Over the years, despite her Mom's sincere attempts to stop it from happening, Kelly did, in fact, follow her Mom's mom's path, except she could not handle the strict rules of these diet programs. She would lose some weight, then eventually quit, feeling more defeated with each attempt. She eventually dieted her way up to 315 pounds and had gastric bypass surgery. She made the changes that the doctor's recommended. Even though she never reached her goal, she did lose 150 pounds, keeping it off several years. As she slowly returned to her old eating habits, she started the inevitable weight regain. Feeling completely defeated that she had failed the ultimate diet solution, Kelly gave up all hope of ever losing weight and being a healthy weight.

Consider this case study through the lens of the wellness habits you have learned so far.

For each wellness habit, analyze the data and answer these questions.

- What evidence of the wellness habit did you observe?
- What would have been different if you had observed more evidence of the wellness habit?
- Considering that every person is responsible for their own choices and behaviors, what advice would you give Kelly moving forward in relation to this wellness habit?

## *Reflection of Analysis*

What were the overall lessons that you took from this case study?

How does this apply to your life? What actions will you take in your life based on the lessons learned from Kelly's story?

## **Reflection and Application*

EXIT SLIP

Jot down what you learned about the wellness habit of positive mindset.

Discuss how incorporating a positive mindset into your life will help you live a healthy lifestyle moving forward. How will doing so help you make a mindset shift?

List at least 5 five actions that you will incorporate into your life on a regular basis to enable a positive mindset to become an automatic wellness habit in your life.

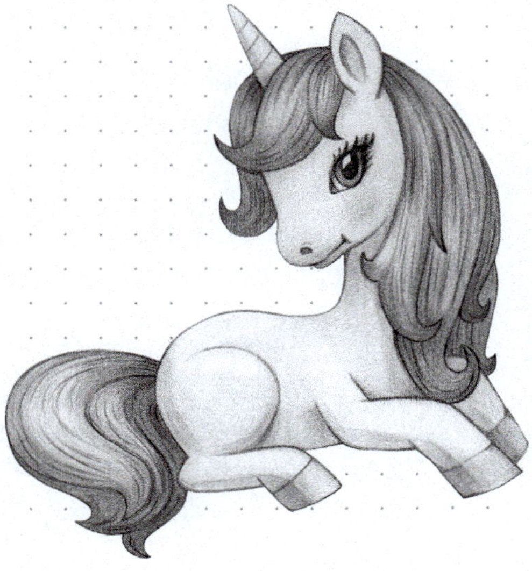

# WEEK 5 FOCUS:
# Wellness Habit: Joyful Activity

There are many limiting beliefs regarding movement and exercise that are likely holding you back from finding joy in incorporating movement in your day. It is time to become aware of them!

- If you're not sweating, you're not doing any good.
- Exercise is punishment for eating bad food.
- Exercise is a chore.
- Exercise is boring!
- If I eat something I shouldn't have, or too much of something, I must work it off through exercise.
- Exercise is only for young people.
- I must join a gym to exercise, and I can't afford that right now.
- Exercise must be done in one big chunk of time.
- I don't have time to exercise.

You have learned that limiting beliefs are false statements. Now, look back through these limiting beliefs and state the truth. It is going to be the opposite of what is written.

Even the word exercise evokes negative emotions for many people, like bad memories of gym class in school or being forced to play games and participate in sports that you did not enjoy.

And there is a big clue to the problem of "...being forced to play games and participate in sports that you did not enjoy." At that time, you had no free will or sense of empowerment to decide what most suited you.

Likely, after school and over the weekend, you were out playing with your friends, doing things you loved, and no-one had to make you do it. You just did what was fun and did not think about it being "exercise".

So, let's ditch that word. Some people love to go hard, work up a sweat, feel the burn, and continually beat their own personal bests. For them, that is the true essence of joyful movement. It is what they love to do.!

For another person, this same regimen might be torture. A gentle walk while listening to great music or podcasts is a joyful activity for this person.

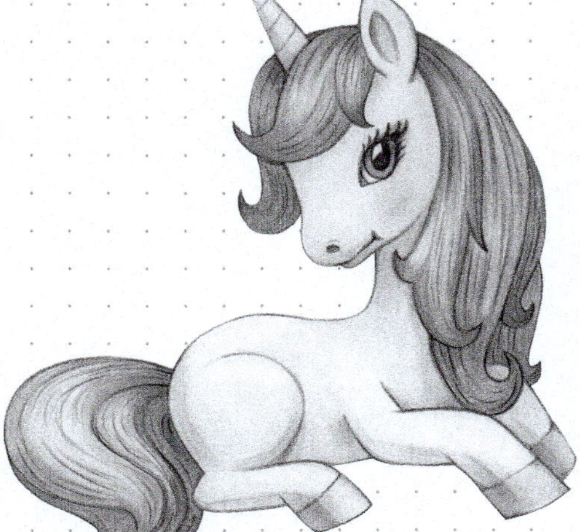

Finding a way to integrate enjoyable movement into your day is important for your overall health and wellness. It promotes stress reduction, mental clarity, heart health, and helping prevent future disease.

What joyful movement means to you is personal and will be different for each of us.

Many of us say we hate exercise. However, when asked to think of what they loved to do as a child or what kind of play they engaged in with their friends, adults always animatedly speak of their great childhood and all of the fun they had.

Bike riding often comes up, as does swimming, running, climbing trees, playing informal sports games with the neighborhood gang, and hiking. Many have fond memories of various movement activities; they just do not think of them as exercise. They were just play!

It is time to play again. Think back on your own childhood to point you in the right direction. Were you more of a team-oriented kid, or did you enjoy solo activities?

Be open to new ideas! Try a kickboxing class, yoga, tai chi, swimming laps, water aerobics, or chair yoga. Maybe doing 18 holes gets your juices flowing?

Or are you more practically minded? Do you love doing some serious cleaning, including washing walls and hosing down patios? Do gardening, mowing, trimming, and raking leaves in your yard fit the bill?

Do you love to run and play with your grandchildren?

All these things can be joyful movement if they are things you truly enjoy. Movement does not have to mean a sport or involve dumbbells. Just keep looking until you find movement to incorporate into your life that invigorates and energizes you, something you look forward to. It exists!

Ultimately, you are empowered to be in charge of your own health, and finding movement you enjoy is your responsibility. So have fun as you solve this puzzle for yourself.

Continue to cultivate a positive mindset and approach your search with a sense of wonder and excitement. If you try something and do not enjoy it, no big deal. Keep experimenting! The only way you will fail is if you give up.

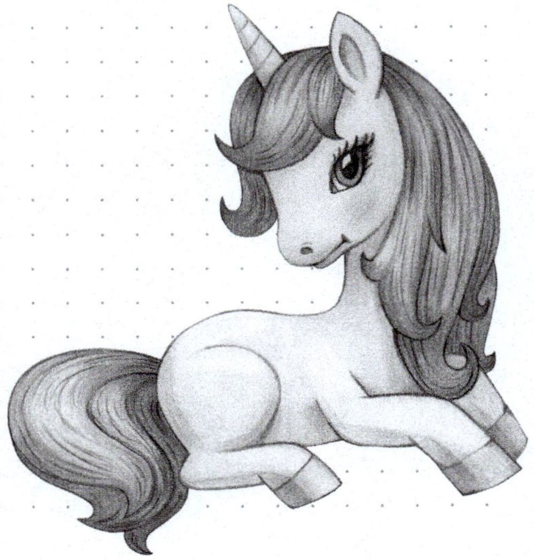

## **Activity Selections & and Scheduling*

Select activities to reinforce the new wellness habit and schedule them into your week. Be thoughtful and intentional as you participate in them. The more effort and thought you put into the activities, the more you will benefit from them.

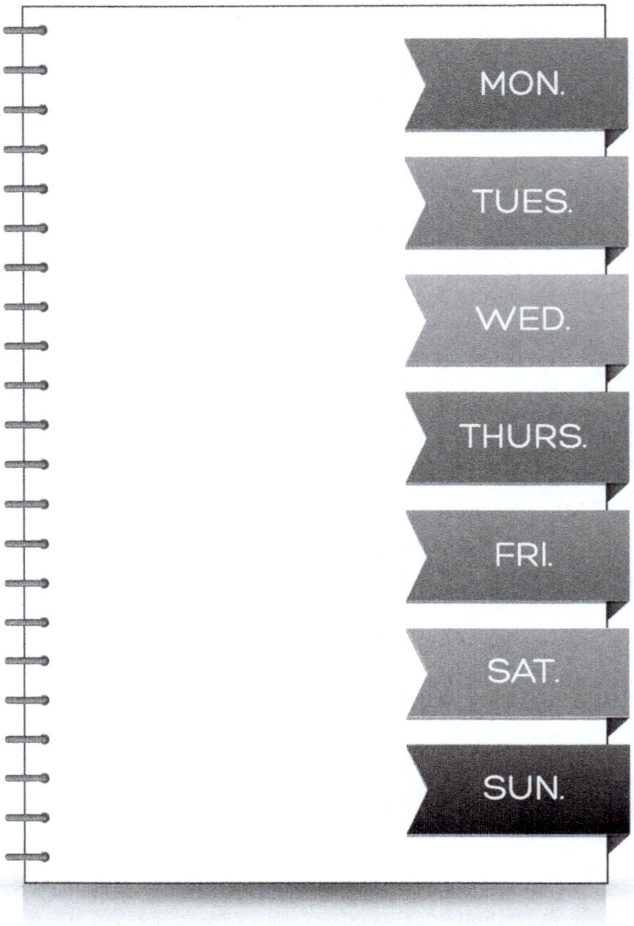


## *Activity Selection*

PRO/CON GRID

Brainstorm a list of 5 five movement activities that you might realistically choose to participate in. For each activity, list the pros of participating in this activity, and the cons of doing it.

Review your work. How many of the activities sound fun, and you are willing to try? If you cannot come up with 3, go back to the drawing board with another 5 five activities and try it again.

Continue this exercise until you have 3 three solid activities that you are willing to try. Then schedule time into your week and give them a go! You can introduce one activity per week or go for two or even three. You are in charge, so it is totally up to you!

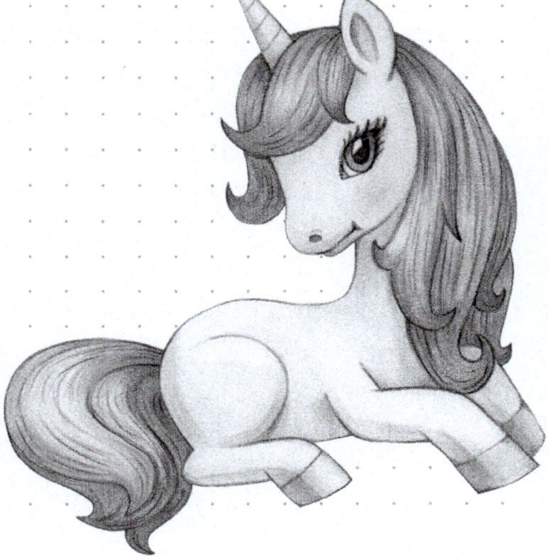

## *Activity Selection*

TEMPTING TIMELINE

Create a timeline.

At the left on the timeline, draw illustrations of you participating in your favorite movement activities. Begin with your earliest memory of something that you really had fun doing. Continue your timeline as you got older and grew into different movement activities that you loved. Keep the timeline going into your high school and then post-high school years.

Now review your timeline. Do you see any common themes? Identify 5 activities that you loved through the years that you are tempted to begin experimenting with. Either the specific activity, or an activity that resembles it, in adult form. Capture the sense of fun, and consider how you can recreate that feeling.

For example, if you adored climbing trees, is there a gym close to you with a climbing wall? If not, how else can you somehow incorporate climbing into your life? Be creative and look for ways to bring those fun childhood activities to life.

## *Activity Selection*

CREATIVE COLLAGE

Create a photo collage of all the physical activities that you would love to do if you had no weight and/or other physical limitations.

It can either be a video collage, or you can cut out magazine pictures and create your own masterpiece to motivate yourself.

Come back to your photo collage often for inspiration and motivation!

## **Pulling it All Together: Make it Personal*

Write your own personal journey, that brought you to this point in your life. Model it after Kelly's case study. It can be any length you like.

Next, map or outline what you were thinking, feeling, and doing as you review your personal journey/case study.

Finally, think about what you have learned through your work these last five weeks. Imagine what your life will look like as you empower yourself to utilize the five wellness habits. Envision what your life will look like as you incorporate these habits:

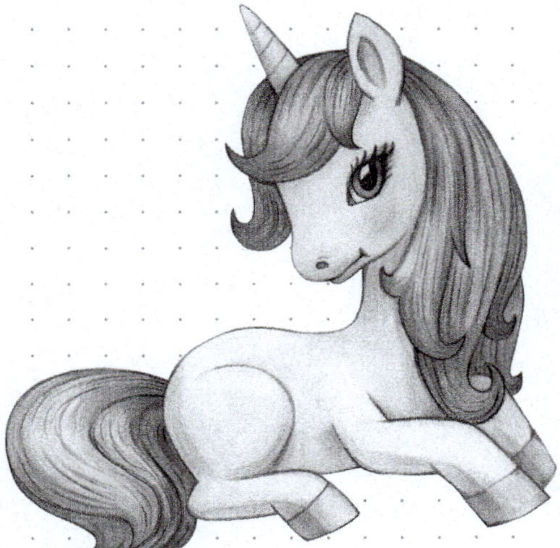

1. Self-Love and Self-Acceptance
2. Empowered Thinking
3. Self Honoring Choices
4. Positive Mindset
5. Joyful Movement

Map this journey as you do things differently and achieve a different outcome. This map can look however you want it to look. It can take the form of an essay. Write a song or a poem to show what you believe your new outcome is going to be. It can be a painting or drawing, or another creative endeavor. It can be anything you want it to be, because, as always, you are empowered to write your own ending!

PART THREE

# Fast with Paige "PLUS"

# Resources to Fuel Your Empowerment and Success

**Woman's World Cover*

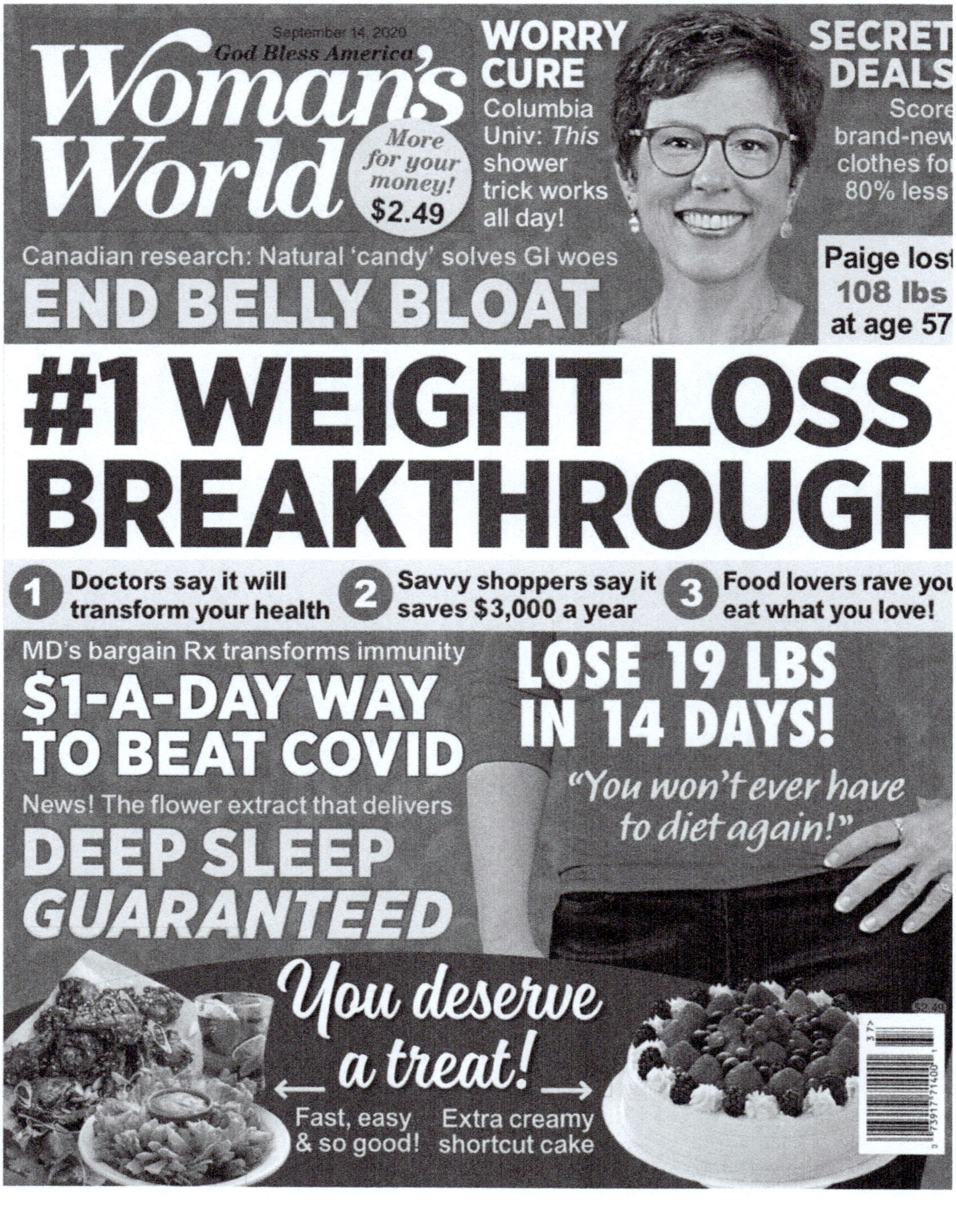


I was honored to be selected by Woman's World magazine, from among many intermittent fasting success stories submitted from across the United States, to be the focus of their story on IF.

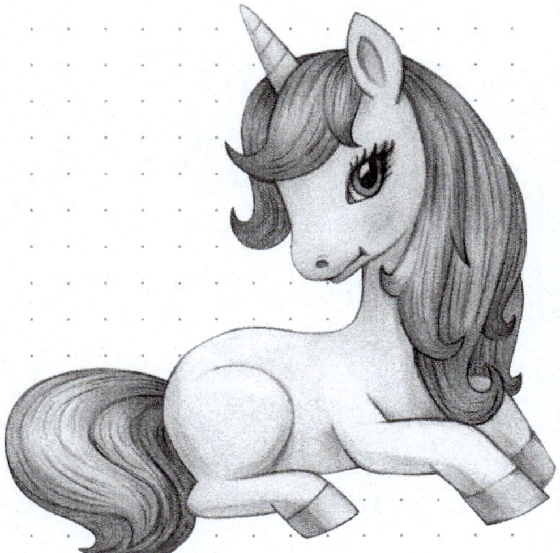

# What is a "Clean Fast"?

**Yes!**

* Water (*unflavored*)
* Black coffee (*unflavored*)
* Any plain tea brewed from actual dried tea leaves only (*black tea, green tea, etc., unflavored varieties only*)
* Mineral water, club soda, sparkling water, or seltzer water (*unflavored*)
* Minerals/electrolytes/salt (*with no additives/flavors*)
* Medications, as prescribed by your health care provider

**Maybe...**

*We call this the "grey area"*

* Peppermint essential oil for breath freshening only, NOT for water-enhancing (*select food-grade and use sparingly*)
* Herbal tea with a bitter flavor profile
* Vitamins and supplements (*There is no easy answer for all vitamins and supplements. Any that are clearly food-like or listed in the "No" column should be taken within your eating window.*)

**No!**

* Food
* Flavored water
* Flavored coffee
* Fruity, sweet, or matcha teas
* Diet sodas
* Natural or artificial flavors
* Natural or artificial sweeteners
* Gum or mints
* Food-like flavors of any type (*fruit juices, fruit flavors, etc.*)
* Bone broth, broth, or bouillon
* Added fats, including coconut oil, MCT oil, butter, etc.
* Cream, creamers, milk (*of any amount or type*)
* Supplements such as collagen, pre-workouts, BCAAs, exogenous ketones, etc.

When living an intermittent fasting lifestyle, the real magic happens during the clean fast!

*For a full explanation and the science behind these recommendations, visit:*
http://www.ginstephens.com/all-blog-posts/does-a-clean-fast-really-matter

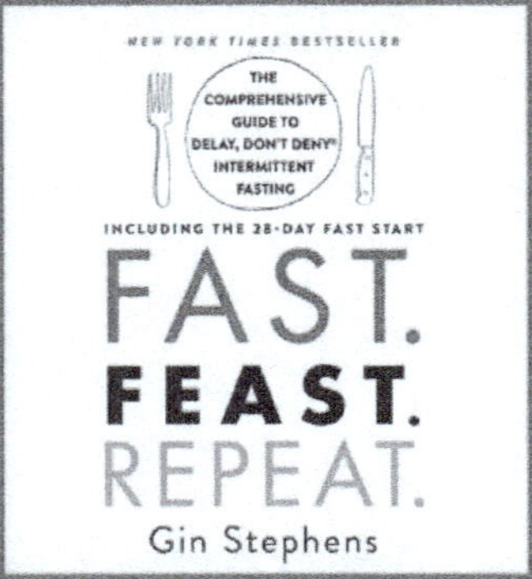


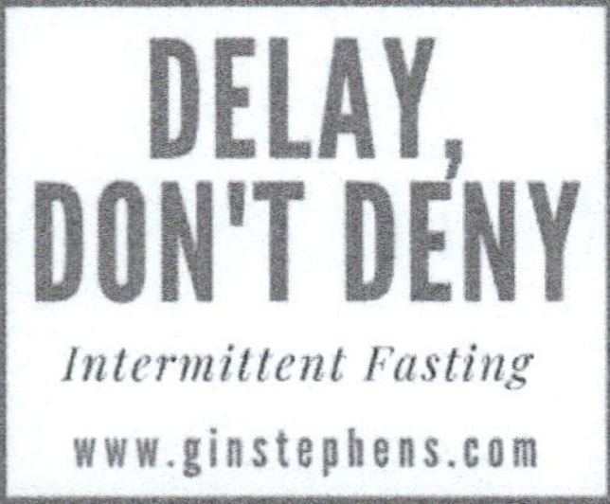


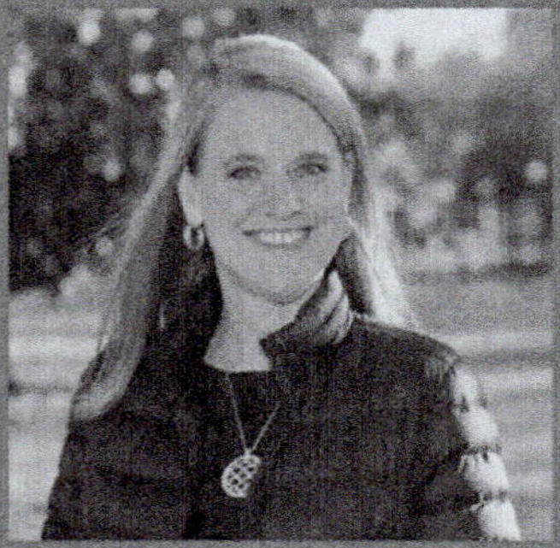

## *Your Wellness Toolkit

Each of us has our own personal wellness toolkit. Our toolkit consists of strategies, actions, and resources we can pull out and use as needed as we work toward achieving our health and weight-loss goals.

As you have learned, daily clean fasting is a strategy that we use with intention. So is eating your food within a daily window. Changing your fasting time and/or your eating window time are tools that you can utilize, if you find that you need to make tweaks to your IF lifestyle. This workbook is full of tools and strategies that we have access to anytime we need or want to use them.

Fill your toolkit with ideas and strategies that you can use as you need them. The fuller your toolkit, the more likely you are to find the exact strategy or tool when you need it most!

Continue working on empowering yourself to live your best and healthiest life! These resources will help you continue learning, and information is power. Feeling powerful is fuel to reinforce your permanent mindset and lifestyle shift, allowing you to experience lifelong success.

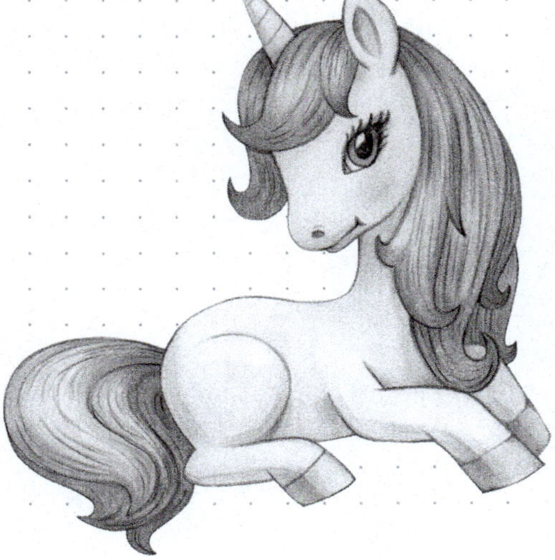

## *Books*

Delay, Don't Deny. Gin Stephens, PhD

Fast. Feast. Repeat. Gin Stephens, PhD

Feast Without Fear Gin Stephens, PhD

AC: The Power of Appetite Correction Bert Herring, MD

Atomic Habits James Clear

The Obesity Code Jason Fung, MD

The Diabetes Code Jason Fung, MD

Unbelievable Freedom: How We Transformed Our Health

and Happiness With Intermittent Fasting Ryan & Kim Smith

Unmired Kim Smith

Lies My Doctor Told Me:

Medical Myths That Can Harm Your Health Ken D. Berry, MD, FAAFP

## *Podcasts*

Listening to podcasts is an entertaining way to stay informed, motivated, and inspired.

Intermittent Fasting Stories
Host: Gin Stephens (I am episode #82) — Available on Himalaya

The Fasting Highway
Host: Graeme Curry (I am Episode #23) — Available on Spotify

The Unbelievable Freedom Podcast
Host: Kim Smith — Available on Himalaya

Living Your Big Bold Life
Host: Bett Lucas — Available on Himalaya

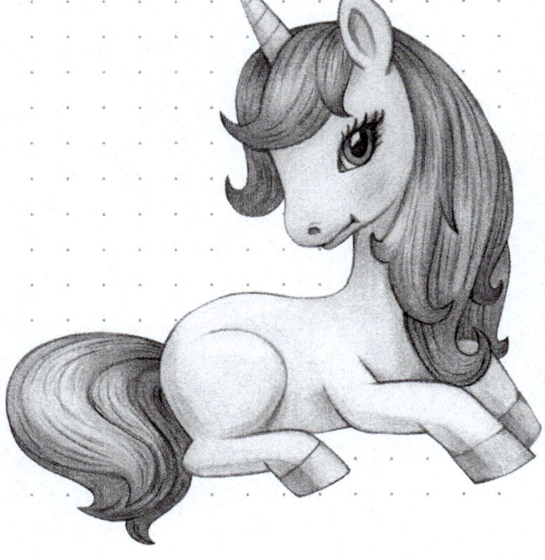

## *Facebook Support Pages/Groups*

"One of the most effective things you can do to build better habits is to join a culture where your desired behavior is the normal behavior." ...James Clear, Atomic Habits

The Fasting PAIGE (Facebook page)

Measure Me L*IF*E (the group includes a web page at measuremelife.com, along with a private Facebook support group featuring a weekly Facebook Live event, a YouTube channel at www.YouTube.com/MeasureMeLife, and a monthly in-person meeting for those in the Louisville, Kentucky, region

Delay, Don't Deny: Intermittent Fasting Support (Facebook Group)

Your Best L{IF}E (Facebook Group)

Delay, Don't Deny: Senior Ladies 60+ (Facebook Group)

The Fasting Highway (Facebook Group)

Fasting Rox (Facebook group)

My Daily Bread of L(IF)E – Christian Intermittent Fasting Support

Motivate with My Betty Lu – Mix of intermittent fasting support along with family and career insights

IF is Life – includes face-to-face meetings for those in the Gilla Valley region of AZ

To continue your journey with me, find information about my coaching and programs at:

www.fastwithpaige.com

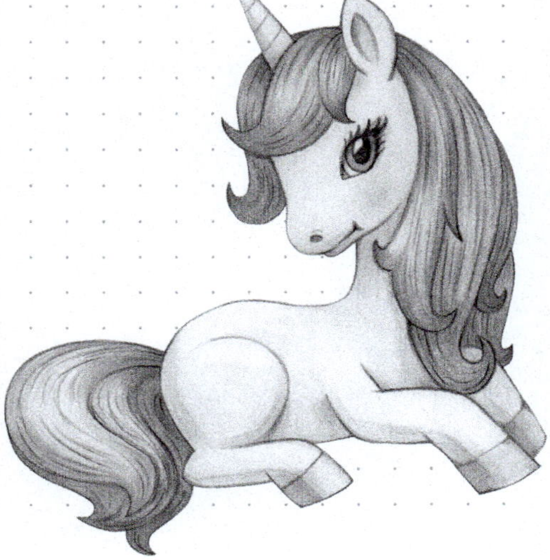

# The Unbelievable Freedom Habit Guide Series

If you enjoyed this book and would like to continue your Unbelievable Freedom journey, there are other titles to collect!

*Fasting Feasting Freedom: A 33 Day Habit Creation Guide* by Kim Smith

*Poster Girl Habits: Creating an Intentional Contentment Practice* by Kim Smith

*A Superhero You: Activate Your Unstoppable Powers* by Barbara Anne Cookson

*Embracing Next: An Empty Nest Enjoyment Guide* by Kim Smith

*The Flow Lane: Creating Life One Thought At A Time* by Lynn M Robinson

*Script A New Life: A Guide to Lasting Change Creation* by Tam Veilleux

*Stop. Drop. Tap! Emotional Freedom Technique for Confidence & Clarity* by Tam Veilleux

*Fasting is the Foundation. A Real Man's View of Unbelievable Freedom* by Ryan Smith

*Fasting With Fervor* by Susannah Juteau M.SC. RD

*Celebrating Your Vibrant Future* by Laurie Lewis

*Three Birds, One Stone* by Kim Smith

Information about all of these workbook-style Habit Guides can be found at www.unbelievablefreedom.com, along with links to their Amazon listings.

Believe in Unbelievable Freedom
Enjoy Your Life!

Printed in Great Britain
by Amazon

56287985R00054